协和医学院系列规划教材

英汉双语

Histology Atlas
(Guidance to Practice)

组织学彩色图谱
（实习指导）

仇文颖　陈咏梅　钱晓菁　主编

U0218919

中国协和医科大学出版社

北　京

图书在版编目（CIP）数据

组织学彩色图谱：实习指导 / 仇文颖，陈咏梅，钱晓菁主编. —北京：中国协和医科大学出版社，2021.8（2024.7重印）.

（协和医学院系列规划教材）

ISBN 978-7-5679-1801-6

Ⅰ.①组… Ⅱ.①仇… ②陈… ③钱… Ⅲ.①人体组织学—图谱 Ⅳ.①R329-64

中国版本图书馆CIP数据核字（2021）第151015号

协和医学院系列规划教材
Histology Atlas（Guidance to Practice）
组织学彩色图谱（实习指导）

主　　编：仇文颖　陈咏梅　钱晓菁
策　　划：马　超
责任编辑：戴申倩　沈紫薇
封面设计：邱晓俐
责任校对：张　麓
责任印制：黄艳霞

出版发行：中国协和医科大学出版社
　　　　　（北京市东城区东单三条9号　邮编100730　电话010-65260431）
网　　址：www.pumcp.com
经　　销：新华书店总店北京发行所
印　　刷：北京建宏印刷有限公司

开　　本：889mm×1194mm　　1/16
印　　张：11.5
字　　数：320千字
版　　次：2021年8月第1版
印　　次：2024年7月第4次印刷
定　　价：68.00元

ISBN 978-7-5679-1801-6

前 言

组织学是医学生必修的核心基础医学课程，是研究人体在光学显微镜下微细结构和电子显微镜下超微结构及其相关功能的科学。教学目标是使学生获得有关人体微细结构的基础理论、基本知识、基本技能，如准确识别各种细胞、组织和器官的结构及了解其与功能的关系，从而为学习生理学、病理学等其他基础医学与临床医学各学科课程奠定基础。课程的核心是掌握其"形"，但对于初涉形态学的学生来说，观察镜下结构还需要较为详细的指导。

北京协和医学院八年制临床医学专业的组织学课程要求观察100余幅各类切片，教学内容较多，包括特殊部位（如鼻中隔）的切片以及特殊染色等，每一幅切片观察重点不同，有些结构比较难以辨别，学生课上时间有限，课下难以获得系统而准确的指导。鉴于此，我们以组织胚胎学教研室多年传承的组织学切片以及编纂的英文实习指导为基础，结合教学目标，编写本实习指导教材。

本教材共计17章，第1～6章为基本组织部分，特殊结缔组织（软骨和骨、血液和血细胞发生单独成章）；第7～17章为各个系统相应章节，以器官为序，描述其基本结构。每一章节均明确了实验教学目标，删减了部分理论课内容，强化了对切片的观察方法，对结构形态特征的描述，配以高清晰度图片，以便于学生掌握。章节最后增设了"问题"版块，引导学生有目的地观察切片。教材中切片编号由章名的英文首字母或缩写加切片顺序来命名，与本校学生实体切片编号保持一致；示教切片为教师课堂展示切片。

本教材文字采用了英汉对照，通过对术语双语的掌握，可以为后续学习其他基础与临床医学课程打下坚实的基础。本教材可作为图谱和实习指导，供临床医学及相关专业学生、青年教师学习组织学使用。

感谢北京协和医学院教学改革项目的支持，本教材得以立项并正式出版。在编写过程中部分图片的切片制备得到了我校郭燕和徐园园老师的帮助；乌正赉和蒋育红老师在英文审校上给予了专业指导，在此一并表示感谢！由于作者水平有限，本教材中可能存在不当之处，望读者能在学习、教学中给予批评指正。

仇文颖　陈咏梅　钱晓菁
北京协和医学院

目　录

Chapter 1　EPITHELIAL TISSUE
第一章　上皮组织

Teaching and Learning Objectives

- To understand the principle for classification of epithelial tissue.
- To identify the features and distribution of different types of epithelia.
- To identify specific structure of epithelial cell surface: microvilli, cilia, cellular junctional complexes and basement membrane.

教学目标

- 掌握上皮组织分类原则。
- 辨认不同类型上皮特征，掌握其分布。
- 辨认上皮细胞表面的特殊结构：微绒毛、纤毛、细胞连接复合体、基膜。

1.Simple squamous epithelium

This slide shows a surface view of the mesentery from frog in whole mount. The cellular limit (or delineation) appears black (or dark) with AgNO₃ stain. Polygonal cell body and curved cellular juncture can be seen in epithelial cells, with centrally located nucleus by counter-staining method (Fig. 1-1).

1.单层扁平上皮

此张切片为蛙肠系膜铺片表面观，通过硝酸银染色勾勒出黑色细胞界限。可见上皮细胞为多边形，细胞交界曲折，复染的细胞核居中（图1-1）。

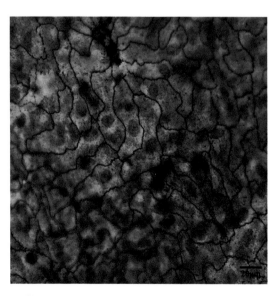

Fig. 1-1　Simple squamous epithelium, mesentery, whole mount, by AgNO₃ stain (slide No. E2)

图1-1　单层扁平上皮，肠系膜铺片，硝酸银染色（切片 No. E2）

2.Simple squamous epithelium and simple cuboidal epithelia

Under microscope with low-power objective lens, try to distinguish lighter stain medulla from darker stain cortex, identifiable with round renal corpuscle in the cortex. Observing renal capsule around renal corpuscles under microscope with high-power objective lens, try to distinguish simple squamous epithelium lining renal capsule, where nucleus bulges into the lumen with difficultly distinguishable flattened cytoplasm. Cross-sections of the closely packed renal tubules can be found in this section. Surface of most renal tubules lines with simple cuboidal epithelium, with centrally-located spherical nuclei, which can be identified as cuboidal in nature with basically equal height and width of its cytoplasm even its cellular limit not so clear. There are blood vessels in the renal interstitium, which lined with simple squamous epithelium referred to endothelium, whereas red blood cells within their lumen are helpful for their identification (Fig. 1-2).

2.单层扁平上皮与单层立方上皮

低倍镜下区别染色稍浅的髓质和染色稍深的皮质，皮质中圆形肾小体有助于辨认。高倍镜下观察肾小体外圈的肾小囊，辨认肾小囊被覆的单层扁平上皮：细胞核凸向管腔，胞质扁平而难以辨认。切片可见密集排列的肾小管截面。多数肾小管表面被覆的单层立方上皮特征如下：细胞核圆，居中，即使细胞界限不清，也可通过胞质长宽基本相等的特征辨认出细胞属立方形态。肾间质中分布有血管，血管腔面被覆有单层扁平上皮，又称内皮，管腔内的红细胞有助于辨认血管（图1-2）。

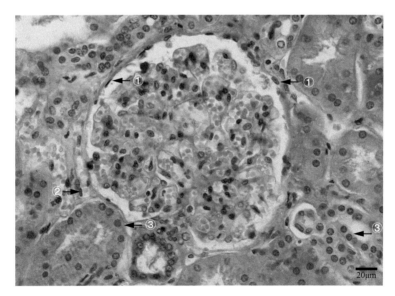

Fig. 1-2 Simple squamous epithelium and simple cuboidal epithelium, kidney, by H.E. stain (slide No. Ur1)

图1-2 单层扁平上皮与单层立方上皮，肾，HE染色（切片No. Ur1）

①simple squamous epithelium of renal capsule
②endothelium of blood vessel
③simple cuboidal epithelium of renal tubule

①肾小囊单层扁平上皮
②血管内皮
③肾小管单层立方上皮

3.Simple columnar epithelium

Plicae circulares projecting into jejunal lumen and intestinal villi, which are covered with simple columnar epithelium, can be seen in one aspect of the section under microscope with low-power objective. Under high power objective, densely-packed columnar epithelial cells can be seen, with elongated nucleus located at base. Broader acidophilic stripe can be seen at cell free surface, referred to striated border, a structure with densely-lined microvilli (Fig. 1-3). (Note that in oblique section, epithelial cells may appear multilayered nucleate in nature.) Specialized unicellular gland among columnar epithelial cells can be seen, i.e., goblet cell, with cytoplasm stained pale, wine-cup in shape and dark triangular nucleus located close to the base. Observing simple columnar epithelium in jejunal villi with oil-immersion objective, the structure of dark stain dots can be seen in the lateral surface of columnar epithelial cells (close to their free surface), known as termi-nal bar (Fig. 1-4), i.e., cellular junctional complexes under light microscope.

3.单层柱状上皮

低倍镜下切片一侧可见突入肠腔的环形皱襞及小肠绒毛，绒毛表面覆盖单层柱状上皮。高倍镜下可见柱状上皮细胞紧密排列，细胞核长椭圆形，位于上皮细胞基底。细胞游离面可见较宽的嗜酸性条纹，称纹状缘，为密集排列的整齐的微绒毛结构（图1-3）。（注意：斜切的上皮细胞可呈现多层细胞核。）柱状上皮细胞间有特化的单细胞腺——杯状细胞，细胞染色浅淡，呈高脚杯状，细胞核深染，呈三角形，靠近基底。油镜观察空肠绒毛单层柱状上皮，柱状上皮细胞侧面（靠近游离面）可见深染点状结构，称闭锁堤或终棒（图1-4），为光镜下见到的细胞连接复合体。

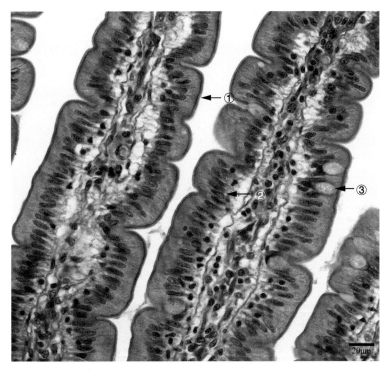

20μm

Fig. 1-3   Simple columnar epithelium, jejunum, by H.E. stain (slide No. DT8)

图 1-3   单层柱状上皮，空肠，HE染色（切片 No. DT8）

①striated border　　　　　　　　①纹状缘

②columnar epithelial cell　　　　②柱状上皮细胞

③goblet cell　　　　　　　　　　③杯状细胞

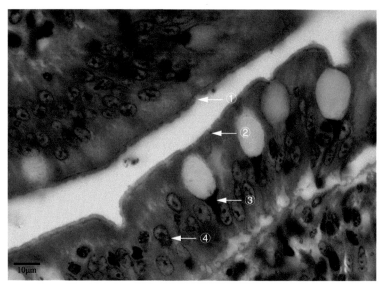

Fig. 1-4　Terminal bar, jejunum, by I.H. stain (demonstration slide)
图1-4　闭锁堤，空肠，铁苏木素染色（示教切片）

①striated border　　　　　　　　①纹状缘
②terminal bar　　　　　　　　　②闭锁堤
③goblet cell　　　　　　　　　　③杯状细胞
④columnar epithelial cell　　　　④柱状上皮细胞

Basement membrane locates at the basal surface of epithelium, where reticular fibers appear as black threads by AgNO$_3$ stain (Fig. 1-5).

基底膜位于上皮组织基底面，其含有的网状纤维在银染下呈黑色细线状（图1-5）。

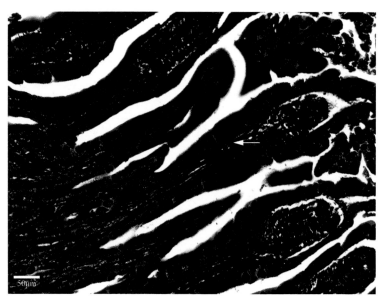

Fig. 1-5　Basement membrane, jejunum, by AgNO$_3$ stain (demonstration slide)
图1-5　基底膜，空肠，硝酸银染色（示教切片）

4.Pseudostratified ciliated columnar epithelium

Observing under low power objective, pseudostratified ciliated columnar epithelium is stronger basophilic in nature than other tissue in this slide. Observing characteristic epithelium in respiratory system with high power objective, pseudostratified ciliated columnar epithelium can be seen, characterized by irregularly distributed nuclei. Those with elongated oval nuclei and loose chromatin, located close to the surface in cross-section are nuclei of ciliated cells, and those with small-sized, round, dark nuclei located near epithelial basement membrane are nuclei of basal cells. Goblet cells can be seen among ciliated cells, with their body size smaller than those in small intestine. At the free (or apical) surface of this epithelium, specialized projections, known as cilia, can be clearly seen (Fig. 1-6).

4.假复层纤毛柱状上皮

低倍镜观察切片，嗜碱性较强的一侧为上皮组织。高倍镜观察呼吸道特征性上皮，假复层纤毛柱状上皮特点：横切面上可见不规则分布的细胞核，其中长椭圆形、染色质疏松、位置较高的为纤毛细胞细胞核；靠近基底面，体积小、圆形、深染核的为基底细胞细胞核；纤毛细胞间可见杯状细胞，其体积小于肠道内的杯状细胞。上皮游离面纤毛清晰可见（图1-6）。

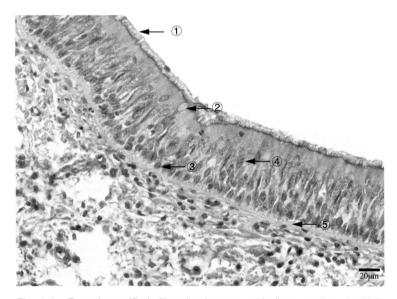

Fig. 1-6　Pseudostratified ciliated columnar epithelium, trachea, by H.E. stain (slide No. Re2)

图1-6　假复层纤毛柱状上皮，气管，HE染色（切片No. Re2）

①cilia　　　　　　　　　　　①纤毛
②goblet cell　　　　　　　　②杯状细胞
③basal cell　　　　　　　　③基底细胞
④ciliated cell　　　　　　　④纤毛细胞
⑤basement membrane　　　⑤基膜

5.Stratified squamous epithelium

Esophageal lumen is lined with non-keratinized stratified squamous epithelium, resting on uneven basement membrane. Connective tissue appearing papilla-like projection into the epithelium can be seen. That close to basement membrane is basal cell layer, with smaller and round nuclei, stronger basophilic cytoplasm, occasionally mitosis can be seen, that associated with epithelial renewal. Cells in the intermediate layer present polyhedral in shape, with clear intercellular boundary, round and centrally-located nuclei, the closer to the free surface they are, the more flattened they become, with smaller, darker and flat nucleus. Cells on the outermost layers consist of thin squamous epithelial cells, with flattened and dark-stain nuclei (Fig. 1-7).

5. 复层扁平上皮

食管腔面被覆有未角化的复层扁平上皮：基底面坐落于凹凸不平的基膜上，可见结缔组织呈乳头状突入上皮；紧贴基膜的为基底细胞层，核小而圆，胞质嗜碱性较强，偶尔可见有丝分裂像，与上皮更新有关；中间层细胞呈多边形，细胞界限清楚，胞核圆、居中，越接近表层，细胞越扁平；最表层细胞为扁平的鳞状细胞，核扁，较小，染色深（图1-7）。

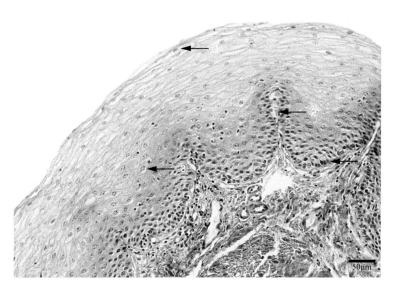

Fig. 1-7　Stratified squamous epithelium, esophagus, by H.E. stain (slide No. DT4)

图1-7　复层扁平上皮，食管，HE染色（切片No. DT4）

①superficial layer cell
②papilla of connective tissue
③intermediate layer cell
④basal layer cell

①表层细胞
②结缔组织乳头
③中间层细胞
④基底层细胞

6.Transitional epithelium

This is a section prepared from a contracted bladder. Stratified nuclei can be seen in the epithelium, with larger cuboidal cells in the outermost layer, acidophilic cytoplasm, round and centrally-located nuclei. These cells projecting towards the lumen are also called "dome cells". Cells in the intermediate layer present polyhedral in shape, with the deepest cells appearing cuboidal or short-columnar in nature (Fig. 1-8). Morphology and number of stratum of epithelial cells vary with the status of urinary bladder distension, so referred to transitional epithelium (Fig. 1-9).

6.变移上皮

此切片为收缩状态的膀胱。上皮内可见多层细胞核，最表层细胞呈大立方形，胞质嗜酸性，胞核圆、居中，细胞凸向腔面，又称盖细胞。中间层细胞呈多边形，最深处细胞为立方或矮柱状（图1-8）。随膀胱充盈状态不同，细胞形态及层数均可变化，故称变移上皮（又称移行上皮）（图1-9）。

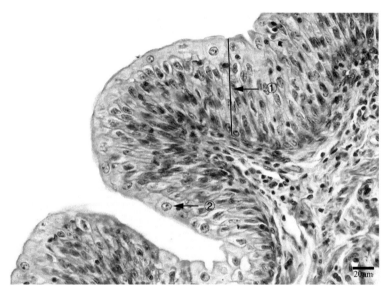

Fig. 1-8   Transitional epithelium, urinary bladder, by H.E. stain (slide No. Ur3)

图1-8　变移上皮，膀胱，HE染色（切片No. Ur3）

①transitional epithelium in contracted bladder
②dome cell

①收缩状态膀胱中的变移上皮
②盖细胞

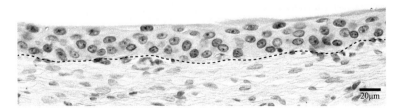

Fig. 1-9   Transitional epithelium in distended bladder (demonstration slide)

图1-9　扩张状态膀胱变移上皮（示教切片）

Number of cell layer reduced and cells flattened especially in superficial layer.

变移上皮细胞层数变少，细胞形态扁平，尤其是表层细胞。

Questions	问题
How can you distinguish the stratified squamous epithelium from transitional epithelium in the distended bladder?	如何区分复层扁平上皮与扩张膀胱中的变移上皮？

Chapter 2　CONNECTIVE TISSUE
第二章　结缔组织

Teaching and Learning Objectives

- To identify morphological characteristics of fibroblasts, and to understand morphological difference between their active and silent status.
- To identify morphological characteristics of macrophages, mast cells, plasma cells and adipocytes.
- To identify morphological characteristics of collagenous fibers, elastic fibers and reticular fibers with special (or specific) staining.
- To distinguish varied types of connective tissue based on the proportions of fibers, stroma, and cells that they account for.

教学目标

- 辨认成纤维细胞的形态特点，了解其功能活跃和不活跃状态的形态区别。
- 辨认巨噬细胞、肥大细胞、浆细胞、脂肪细胞的形态特点。
- 辨认胶原纤维、弹性纤维和网状纤维在其特殊染色方法下的不同形态特点。
- 根据纤维（包括类型）、基质和细胞等各种成分占比不同而辨识不同类型的结缔组织。

1.Fibroblasts

Fibroblasts present large and star-shaped, with irregularly fine and long cytoplasmic processes, round or ovoid and pale-stain nuclei, and finely granular chromatin. Nucleolus can be seen, with slightly basophilic cytoplasm. Mitotic cells are frequently seen in this section (Fig. 2-1).

1.成纤维细胞

成纤维细胞呈星形，胞质有很多细长的突起，核圆形或卵圆形，染色较浅，可见核仁，胞质略嗜碱性，常见有丝分裂细胞（图2-1）。

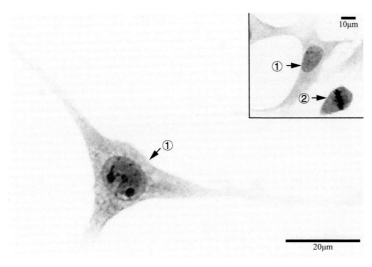

Fig. 2-1　Fibroblasts, cultured fibroblasts, by H.E. stain (slide No. C2)

图2-1　成纤维细胞，培养的成纤维细胞，HE染色（切片No. C2）

①cultured fibroblast　　　①培养的成纤维细胞
②cells at mitotic phase　　②细胞有丝分裂相

2.Loose connective tissue

Trypan blue is injected intraperitoneally to the rats, and mesentery are collected from the rats two days later, and then mounted on the slide for observation under microscope, with resorcin-fuchsin and carmine stain.

Try to observe mainly the following structure in this slide: ①Fibroblasts are the most numerous cells in the preparation, with oval nuclei, very light stain cytoplasm, and hardly distinguishable; ②Nuclei of macrophages are smaller and round in shape, with phagocytosed blue dyes in cytoplasm, easily distinguishable from fibroblasts; ③Collagenous fibers are stained red, appearing long, straight or wavy threads, or ribbon-like in shape, running in varied directions; ④Elastic fibers can be seen as dark purple wavy strands in this preparation (Fig. 2-2).

2.疏松结缔组织

大鼠腹腔内注射台盼蓝，两天后取肠系膜铺片，间苯二酚-复红和胭脂红染色。主要观察以下结构特征：①成纤维细胞是组织中最多的细胞，核卵圆形，胞质染色很浅，几乎不可分辨；②巨噬细胞胞核小而圆，胞质内有吞噬的蓝色染料，很容易与成纤维细胞区别；③胶原纤维较长，染成红色，呈直线、波浪状或带状，多向走行；④弹性纤维染成暗紫色的波浪状细线（图2-2）。

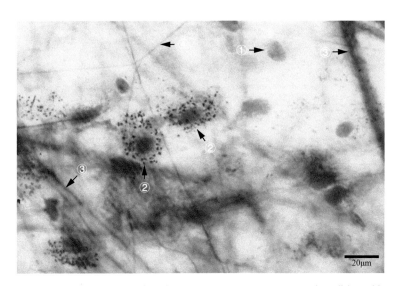

Fig. 2-2　Loose connective tissue, mesentery mount on the slide, with trypan blue intraperitoneal injection and by resorcin-fuchsin and carmine stain (slide No. C1)

图2-2　疏松结缔组织，肠系膜组织铺片，腹腔台盼蓝注射及间苯二酚-复红和胭脂红染色（切片No. C1）

①fibroblast	①成纤维细胞
②macrophage	②巨噬细胞
③collagenous fiber	③胶原纤维
④elastic fiber	④弹性纤维

Mast cell is oval in shape, with smaller nucleus and cytoplasm containing coarse metachromatic purplish-red granules, and disperses in cluster along blood vessels (Fig. 2-3).

肥大细胞卵圆形，核小，胞质中充满粗大的异染性、染成紫红色的颗粒，常常沿血管成群分布（图2-3）。

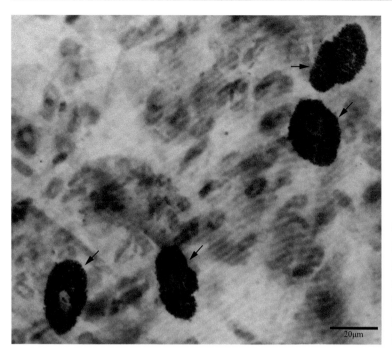

Fig. 2-3　Mast cells, loose connective tissue, mesentery mount on the slide, by resorcin-fuchsin and carmine stain (demonstration slide)

图2-3　肥大细胞，疏松结缔组织，肠系膜组织铺片，间苯二酚－复红和胭脂红染色（示教铺片）

Plasma cell is oval in shape with abundant basophilic cytoplasm, with "clock-faced" nucleus usually situated eccentrically in it (Fig. 2-4).

浆细胞呈卵圆形，胞质嗜碱性，细胞核呈"钟面"样，常偏位（图2-4）。

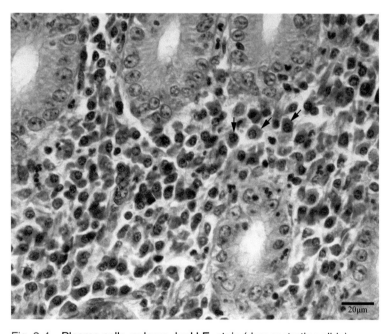

Fig. 2-4　Plasma cells, pylorus, by H.E. stain (demonstration slide)
图2-4　浆细胞，胃幽门，HE染色（示教切片）

Reticular fibers can not be distinguished in H.E. stain, but can be seen only with silver impregnation method, where they appear black strands forming the framework to support lymph nodes (Fig. 2-5).

网状纤维HE染色无法分辨。银染后，呈黑色的细线，构成了淋巴结的支架结构（图2-5）。

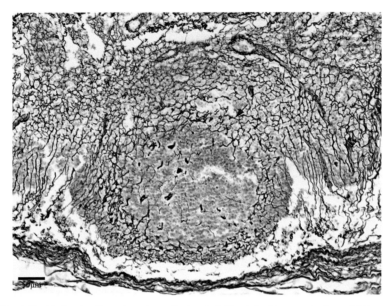

Fig. 2-5　Reticular fiber, lymph node, by AgNO₃ stain (demonstration slide)

图2-5　网状纤维，淋巴结，硝酸银染色（示教切片）

3.Irregular dense connective tissue and adipose tissue

Dermis is composed of irregular dense connective tissue, and numerous irregularly lined collagenous fibers stained red can be seen in the section. Fibroblasts scatter randomly in these collagenous fibers, with dense, dark-stain nuclei. Other connective tissue cells are infrequently seen (Fig. 2-6).

3.不规则致密结缔组织和脂肪组织

真皮由不规则致密结缔组织构成，可见大量不规则排列的胶原纤维，染成红色。成纤维细胞随机散布在胶原纤维之间，胞核致密而染色深。其他结缔组织细胞少见（图2-6）。

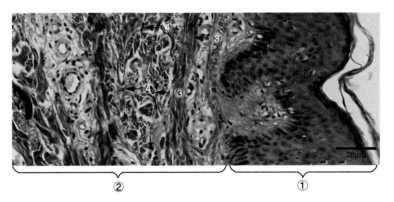

Fig. 2-6　Irregular dense connective tissue, skin, by H.E. stain (slide No. Sk2)

图2-6　不规则致密结缔组织，皮肤，HE染色（切片No. Sk2）

①epidermis	①表皮
②dermis	②真皮
③collagenous fiber	③胶原纤维
④fibroblast	④成纤维细胞

Adipose tissue composed of lots of adipose cells locates in the subcutaneous tissue at the deeper dermis. Lipid droplets in adipose cells are dissolved during the tissue preparation leaving large vacuoles, with their cytoplasm and nuclei squeezed to the edge of cells, known as "signet ring cell" (Fig. 2-7).

真皮深层的皮下组织中有大量脂肪细胞构成的脂肪组织，脂肪细胞内含有的脂滴在制片过程中被溶解，留下一个大空泡，胞质和核被挤压在细胞边缘，称为"印戒细胞"（图2-7）。

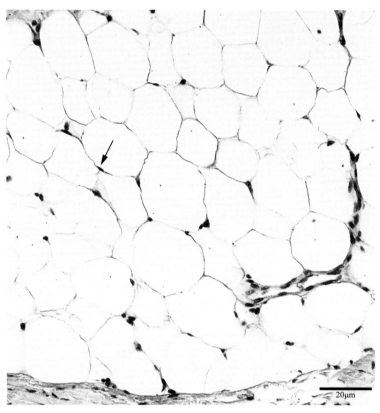

Fig. 2-7　Adipose tissue, skin, by H.E. stain (slide No. Sk2)
图2-7　脂肪组织，皮肤，HE染色（切片No. Sk2）

Arrow: nucleus of adipose cell　　　　　　　　　箭头：脂肪细胞核

4.Regular dense connective tissue
Slide No. C4 and Slide No. C5 are longitudinal and cross section of the tendon, respectively. Note that numerous pink-stain collagenous fibers line regularly in bundles. Fibroblasts lined in rows can be observed among collagenous fiber bundles (Fig. 2-8).

4.规则致密结缔组织
切片No. C4和切片No. C5分别是肌腱的纵切片和横切片。可见大量规则排列的染成红色的胶原纤维束，在胶原纤维束之间可见成列排布的成纤维细胞（图2-8）。

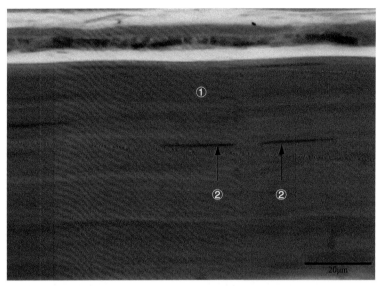

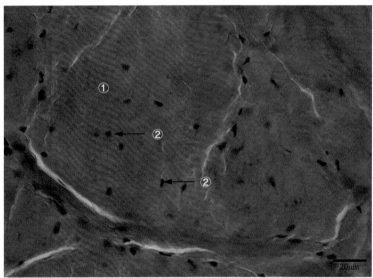

Fig. 2-8　Regular dense connective tissue, tendon, by H.E. stain (slide No. C4, longitudinal section; slide No. C5, cross section)

图2-8　规则的致密结缔组织，肌腱，HE染色（切片No. C4，纵切片；切片No. C5，横切片）

①collagenous fiber　　　　　　　　　①胶原纤维
②fibroblast　　　　　　　　　　　　②成纤维细胞

Questions	问题

How to distinguish collagenous fiber from smooth muscle in the light microscope?

如何在光镜下区分胶原纤维和平滑肌？

Chapter 3　CARTILAGE and BONE

第三章　软骨和骨

Teaching and Learning Objectives

- To identify cartilage and bone, and to distinguish them from other connective tissue.
- To identify basic structures of cartilage in the sections: perichondrium, cartilage matrix, cartilage capsule, fibers, chondrocytes, isogenous groups and cartilage lacunae.
- To distinguish the three types of cartilage: hyaline cartilage, elastic cartilage and fibrocartilage.
- To identify basic structure of bone tissue in the sections: bone matrix and three types of bone cells including osteoblast, osteocyte and osteoclast.
- To identify basic structure of lamellar bone, including osteon, circumferential lamella, interstitial lamella, perforating canal, trabeculae, periosteum and endosteum.
- To describe the processes of two types of osteogenesis, i.e., intramembranous and endochondral bone formation, and to identify the four different regions of epiphyseal plates.

教学目标

- 辨认软骨组织和骨组织，将它们与其他结缔组织区分开。
- 辨认软骨的基本结构（软骨膜、软骨基质、软骨囊、纤维、软骨细胞、同源细胞群和软骨陷窝）。
- 区分3类软骨（透明软骨、弹性软骨和纤维软骨）。
- 辨认骨组织的基本构成成分：骨基质和3种骨细胞（成骨细胞、骨细胞和破骨细胞）。
- 辨认板层骨的基本结构，包括骨单位、环骨板、间骨板、穿通管、骨小梁和骨内、外膜。
- 描述膜内成骨和软骨内成骨两种骨发生的过程，辨认骺板的4个分区。

1.Hyaline cartilage

Slide No. C6 is a cross section of trachea. First, try to find a region that cartilage locate in the slide under microscope with low power objective. Cartilage is wrapped by perichondrium composed of dense connective tissue (with stronger acidophilic). There is no apparent demarcation between perichondrium and its peripheral connective tissue, with chondroblasts in the inner layer of perichondrium and non-distinguishable from fibroblasts at resting cartilage. Cartilage matrix appears weaker basophilic in nature and relatively homogeneous and transparent. Type Ⅱ collagenous fibrils are

1.透明软骨

切片No. C6为气管的横切面，请先用低倍镜找到软骨所在区域。软骨组织被致密结缔组织（具较强嗜酸性）构成的软骨膜包围，软骨膜与周围的结缔组织无明显分界，软骨膜内层有成软骨细胞存在，但处于静息状态的成软骨细胞无法与成纤维细胞区分。软骨基质呈弱嗜碱性，较为均质透明，Ⅱ型胶原原纤维因其直径较细，在光镜下无法分辨。软骨基质中可见大量软骨细胞，靠近软骨膜的软骨细胞较幼稚，多单个分布，细胞呈椭圆形；靠近软骨中央的软骨细胞较圆，胞质多、胞核呈圆形，常

too thin in diameter to be distinguished under light microscope. There are numerous chondrocytes in the cartilage matrix, those close to perichondrium are younger, most appearing solitary in distribution, with round nucleus, and those close to the center of cartilage are more round, with more cytoplasm and round nucleus, and appearing in isogenous groups. The space occupied by chondrocytes in the cartilage matrix is called cartilage lacunae. In preparation of histological slides with paraffin, cytoplasm of chondrocytes shrinks leaving the lacunae visible. Cartilage matrix close to chondrocytes appear stronger basophilic, known as cartilage capsule. There is no blood vessel in the cartilage (Fig. 3-1).

以同源细胞群的形式存在。软骨细胞在基质中所占的空间称为软骨陷窝。制备石蜡切片时，软骨细胞胞质易收缩，使陷窝可见。紧邻软骨细胞的软骨基质呈较强嗜碱性，该区域称为软骨囊。软骨中无血管分布（图3-1）。

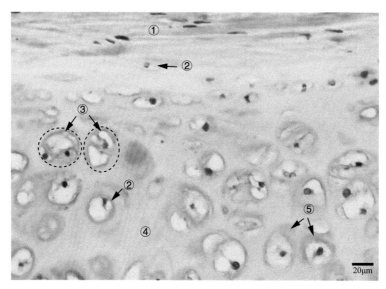

Fig. 3-1　Hyaline cartilage, trachea, by H.E. stain (slide No. C6)
图3-1　透明软骨，气管，HE染色（切片No. C6）

①perichondrium　　　　　　　　　①软骨膜
②chondrocyte　　　　　　　　　　②软骨细胞
③isogenous group　　　　　　　　③同源细胞群
④cartilage matrix　　　　　　　　④软骨基质
⑤cartilage capsule　　　　　　　　⑤软骨囊

2.Elastic cartilage

Slide No. C7 is a cross-section of elastic cartilage from ear pinna, fine thread-like elastic fibers appearing in purplish-red with orcein or resorcin-fuchsin stain can be seen in the cartilage matrix. Note to observe chondrocytes and isogenous groups in elastic cartilage, and to find if there is distinctive difference between elastic cartilage and hyaline cartilage (Fig. 3-2).

2.弹性软骨

切片No. C7为耳郭中的弹性软骨，地衣红或间苯二酚－复红染色后，可见软骨基质中有呈紫红色细线状的弹性纤维存在，请注意观察弹性软骨中软骨细胞、同源细胞群，判断它们是否与透明软骨存在明显差别（图3-2）。

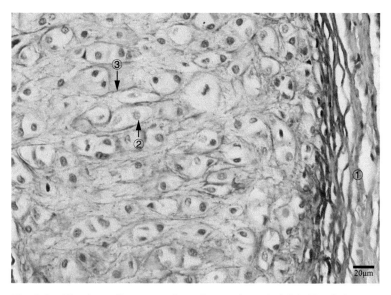

Fig. 3-2   Elastic cartilage, ear pinna, by orcein stain (slide No. C7)
图3-2　弹性软骨，耳郭，地衣红染色（切片No. C7）

①perichondrium　　　　　　　①软骨膜
②chondrocyte　　　　　　　　②软骨细胞
③elastic fibers　　　　　　　　③弹性纤维

3.Fibrocartilage

Slide No. C8 is a longitudinal section of femoral head from a monkey. Try to find fibrocartilage between ligament and articular hyaline cartilage in the slide under microscope with low power objective. There is less ground substance in fibrocartilage, where type Ⅰ collagenous fibers can be apparently seen, with smaller chondrocytes and isogenous groups lined in vertical rows (Fig. 3-3).

3.纤维软骨

切片No. C8为猴股骨头纵切面，请用低倍镜在韧带与关节软骨交界处找到纤维软骨。纤维软骨中无定形基质较少，可见明显的Ⅰ型胶原纤维，软骨细胞较小，同源细胞群的细胞成纵向排列（图3-3）。

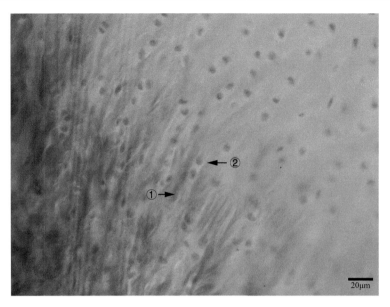

20μm

Fig. 3-3　Fibrocartilage, head of femur, by H.E. stain (slide No. C8)
图3-3　纤维软骨，股骨头，HE染色（切片No. C8）

①type Ⅰ collagenous fiber　　　　①Ⅰ型胶原纤维
②chondrocyte　　　　　　　　　②软骨细胞

4.Ground bone

(1) Femur, by cresyl violet stain

Both cross-section and longitudinal section of adult compact bone can be found in slide No. C10, which has been ground down to a thin wafer, with periosteum and varied bone cells, as well as circumferential lamella, not well preserved during grinding process. Dye stuff can be deposited in various spaces, which can be stained in purplish-blue or black with crystal violet stain.

First try to observe the osteons (Haversian system) on the cross section of ground bone. Osteon is surrounded by cement lines peripherally, with multi-layer concentric bony lamellae around the central canal (Haversian canal) as the center (Fig. 3-4). Among lamellae, lacuna can be found. Observing with high power objective, try to find if there is canaliculi which house the processes of osteocytes. Central canals of the osteons communicate with each other via perforating canal (or Volkmann's canal). The irregular structure composed of multi-layer lamellae among various osteons is called interstitial lamella.

4. 骨磨片

（1）股骨，结晶紫染色

切片No. C10上有成人骨磨片横切、纵切各一块。在骨片磨制的过程中，骨膜和各种骨细胞均脱落，内外环骨板的结构也很难完好保留，结晶紫染色后，染料沉积在各个空腔中，使之呈现蓝紫色或黑色。

先在横切的骨磨片观察骨单位（哈弗斯系统），骨单位的外周有黏合线环绕，中心位置为中央管（哈弗斯管），多层骨板以之为圆心同心圆排列（图3-4）。骨板之间有骨陷窝分布，在高倍镜下观察是否有骨小管（骨细胞突起分布的部位）的存在。各骨单位的中央管可通过穿通管相互联系。在各骨单位之间由多层骨板组成、形态不规则的结构，称为间骨板。

Continue to observe central canal, perforating canal, lamellae and so on in the longitudinal section, and to compare their structural difference between crosssection and longitudinal section.

在纵切的骨磨片上继续观察中央管、穿通管、骨板等，比较横、纵切面上这些结构的差别。

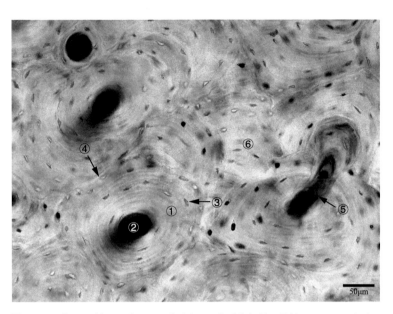

Fig. 3-4   Ground bone, by cresyl violet stain (slide No. C10, cross section)

图3-4   骨磨片，结晶紫染色（切片No. C10，横切片）

① osteon	① 骨单位
② central canal	② 中央管
③ lacuna	③ 骨陷窝
④ cement line	④ 黏合线
⑤ perforating canal	⑤ 穿通管
⑥ interstitial lamella	⑥ 间骨板

(2) Ground bone, by thionine stain

Try to observe the outer circumferential lamellae and the inner circumferential lamellae in the demonstration ground slide (Fig. 3-5). The outer circumferential lamellae are more regular and thicker than the inner circumferential lamellae. Those structures, such as osteons, interstitial lamellae and perforating canals, etc., can also be found in this slide.

（2）骨磨片，硫堇染色

在硫堇染色的骨磨片示教片中观察内环骨板和外环骨板（图3-5）。与内环骨板相比，外环骨板更厚、更规则。内环骨板和外环骨板之间可以观察到骨单位、间骨板和穿通管等结构。

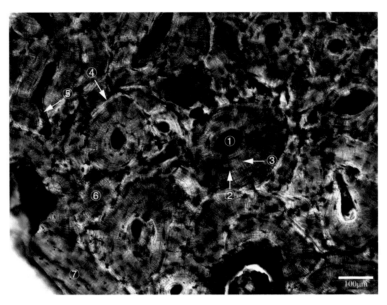

Fig. 3-5　Ground bone, by thionine stain (demonstration slide)

图3-5　骨磨片，硫堇染色（示教切片）

①central canal	①中央管
②lacuna	②骨陷窝
③canaliculi	③骨小管
④cement line	④黏合线
⑤perforating canal	⑤穿通管
⑥interstitial lamella	⑥间骨板
⑦outer circumferential lamellae	⑦外环骨板

5.Decalcified bone

(1) Diaphyses of humerus

Slide No. C9 is a cross-section through the decalcified shaft of the very young humerus. One side of the bone (or osseous) tissue is bone marrow cavity, and the other side are periosteum and skeletal muscle attached to the bone. Note the periosteum is thicke, on the whole, including two distinct layers, the outer layer mainly consists of collagenous fibers served as protective effects, and the inner layer has many osteogenic cells such as osteoprogenitor cells, osteoblasts and so on. The inner side of periosteum is bone tissue, presenting red in H.E. stain due to containing lots of collagenous fibers. The inner and outer circumferential lamellae of the humerus have not completely been formed in the slide. Osteon remodeling varies in degree leading to big difference in the diameter of central canals. Endosteum attaches to the central canal, with blood vessels running within its lumen. The central canal is surrounded by the lamellae concentrically lined, with osteocytes dispersed in the lamella. Irregular interstital lamellae line among the

5.脱钙骨

（1）肱骨骨干

切片No. C9来自幼稚的肱骨骨干，脱钙后制成横切片。骨组织的一侧是骨髓腔，另一侧为骨外膜和骨骼肌。骨外膜较厚，大致可分为两层，外层以纤维为主，起保护作用；内层细胞较多，为骨祖细胞和成骨细胞等。骨外膜内侧为骨组织，因含大量胶原纤维致HE染色呈红色。幼稚的肱骨内环骨板和外环骨板尚未建成，骨单位改建程度也各不相同，导致中央管直径差别较大。中央管内有骨内膜贴附，管腔中可见血管走行。同心圆排列的骨板环绕中央管形成骨单位，每层骨板间有骨细胞分布。骨单位之间有不规则的间骨板分布，除无中央管外其他结构均与骨单位类似（图3-6）。

osteons, with their structure similar to the osteons except
without central canal (Fig. 3-6).

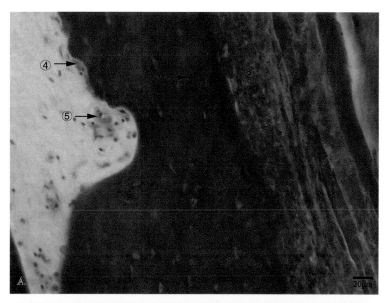

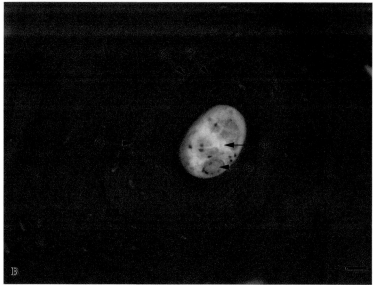

Fig. 3-6　Decalcified bone, by H.E. stain (slide No. C9)
图3-6　脱钙骨，HE染色（切片No. C9）

A.Periosteum and bone tissue	A.骨外膜和骨组织
①outer layer of periosteum	①骨外膜外层
②inner layer of periosteum	②骨外膜内层
③osteocyte	③骨细胞
④endosteum	④骨内膜
⑤blood vessel	⑤血管
B.Compact bone	B.骨密质
①osteon	①骨单位
②osteocyte	②骨细胞
③bone lamella	③骨板
④central canal	④中央管
⑤blood vessel	⑤血管

(2) Perforating fibers (Sharpey fibers)

Coarse and large collagenous fibers that penetrate obliquely through outer circumferential lamellae, known as perforating fibers, which can help tendons or ligaments fixing on the bone (Fig. 3-7). As compared, the perforating fibers from periosteum penetrating through bone tissue are finer and difficult to be observed.

（2）穿通纤维（沙比纤维）

在一些肌腱或韧带固着于骨组织的部位，可见斜穿入外环骨板的较粗大的胶原纤维，称为穿通纤维（图3-7）。与之相比，骨外膜穿入骨组织的穿通纤维则比较细小，不易观察。

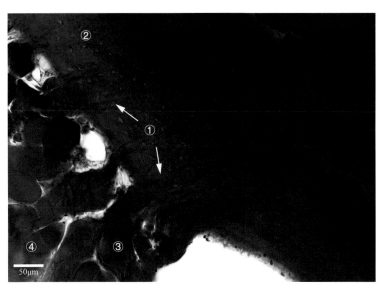

Fig. 3-7　Perforating fibers (Sharpey fibers) , by gold chloride stain (demonstration slide)

图3-7　穿通纤维（沙比纤维），氯化金染色（示教切片）

①perforating fibers
②outer circumferential lamella
③tendon
④skeletal muscles

①穿通纤维
②外环骨板
③肌腱
④骨骼肌

6.Intramembranous ossification

Slide No. C12 shows calvaria in the process of intramembranous ossification, with connective tissue capsule formed by mesenchymal cells in the osteogenic region, and some of the mesenchymal cells differentiate into osteoprogenitor cells and further transfer to osteoblasts beginning to secrete osteoid (or uncalcified bone matrix) and being calcified to form bone. Osteoblasts lined in simple layer can be seen in the surface of irregular bone trabeculae, with stronger basophilic cytoplasm and cuboidal in shape. As in inactivated status, osteoblasts appear flattened in shape. Osteoclasts can be seen scattered in the surface of bone matrix, less in number,

6.膜内成骨

切片No. C12为膜内成骨过程中的顶骨，间充质细胞在将成骨的区域形成结缔组织被膜，其中部分间充质细胞分化成骨祖细胞，进而形成成骨细胞，开始分泌类骨质并钙化成骨。不规则的骨小梁表面可见成骨细胞排列成单层，成骨细胞胞质嗜碱性较强，细胞呈立方形，当其功能不活跃时，呈扁平状。破骨细胞数量较少，散在分布于骨基质表面，其胞质嗜酸性，有多个细胞核。骨基质内可见大量陷于骨陷窝内的骨细胞分布。注意：结缔组织被膜内有丰富的血液供应（图3-8）。

with multinucleated and acidophilic cytoplasm. There are numerous osteocytes that can be seen entrapped in the lacunae of bone matrix. Note the abundant blood supplies in the connective tissue capsule (Fig. 3-8).

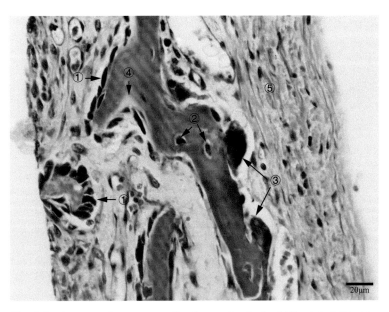

Fig. 3-8   Intramembranous ossification, calvaria, by H.E. stain (slide No. C12)

图3-8   膜内成骨，顶骨，HE染色（切片No. C12）

① osteoblast	① 成骨细胞
② osteocyte	② 骨细胞
③ osteoclast	③ 破骨细胞
④ osteoid	④ 类骨质
⑤ condensed mesenchyme	⑤ 结缔组织被膜

7.Endochondral ossification

(1) Finger

Slide No. C11 is a longitudinal section of finger from a fetus, showing the process of endochondral osteogenesis (Fig. 3-9). In brief, endochondral ossification is a process that first to form a "cartilage model" of the bone at the site of osteogenesis, and then the cartilage tissue degenerates and is replaced by osseous tissue. In the slide, the middle part of cartilage has been replaced by osseous tissue, referred to primary ossification center, with the marrow cavity and irregular trabeculae at the center, the collar of bone as an important support at the periphery, as well as periosteum composed by outer dense connective tissue. Both ends of the cartilage model are still consisted of hyaline cartilage, where sec-

7. 软骨内成骨

（1）手指

切片 No. C11 为胎儿手指的纵切面，可见软骨内成骨的过程（图3-9）。简单地说，软骨内成骨是在将要成骨的部位先形成软骨雏形，之后软骨组织再被骨组织取代的过程。切片中指骨中部软骨组织已经被骨组织取代，此区域被称为初级骨化中心，中央为骨髓腔和不规则的骨小梁，周边是起重要支持作用的骨领，其外侧是致密结缔组织构成的骨外膜。指骨的两端依然为透明软骨，次级骨化中心尚未出现。

ondary ossification center has not yet appeared.

The epiphyseal plate of bone is divided into four zones from cartilage to marrow cavity in proper order: i.e., the resting zone, proliferative zone, hypertrophy and calcified cartilage zone and ossification zone.

The resting zone: consists of hyaline cartilage. The proliferative zone: chondrocytes proliferate rapidly and line in rows along the long axis of the cartilage, with less cytoplasm and dark stain thread-like nuclei. The hypertrophy and calcified cartilage zone: cytoplasm of chondrocytes increases gradually, with nucleus becoming round, then cartilage matrix increased and calcified, and finally the cells get hypertrophy gradually and die. The ossification zone: cartilage cells die, and osteoblasts attach to the surface of calcified cartilage matrix and secrete bone matrix (with stronger acidophilic) and gradually form bone trabeculae as transition, which are digested gradually by osteoclasts and leaving marrow cavity expanded towards both end of the bone.

从软骨向骨髓腔方向骺板依次分为4个区：静止区、增生区、肥大钙化区、骨化区。

静止区：由透明软骨组织构成；增生区：软骨细胞增殖较快，沿软骨长轴成串排列，细胞胞质较少，核呈深染细线状；肥大钙化区：软骨细胞胞质逐渐增多，胞核变圆，随后软骨基质增多并逐渐钙化，细胞逐渐肥大死亡；骨化区：软骨细胞死亡，成骨细胞贴附在钙化的软骨基质表面分泌骨基质（较强嗜酸性），逐渐形成过渡型骨小梁，破骨细胞再不断地消化这些过渡型骨小梁，使骨髓腔向骨两端扩大。

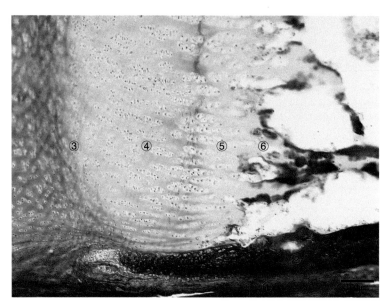

Fig. 3-9　Endochondral ossification, finger, by H.E. stain (slide No. C11)
图3-9　软骨内成骨，手指，HE染色（切片No. C11）

① periosteum	①骨外膜
② bone tissue	②骨组织
③ resting zone	③静止区
④ proliferative zone	④增生区
⑤ hypertrophy and calcified cartilage zone	⑤肥大钙化区
⑥ ossification zone	⑥骨化区

(2) The secondary ossification center

As cartilage grows gradually, the secondary ossification center emerges at the center of cartilage in two expanded ends (Fig. 3-10). Osseous tissue expand continuously all around and replace cartilage tissue, finally keeping articulate and epiphyseal cartilage still in cartilage status. Structure of the secondary ossification is similar to that of the primary ossification center, within which irregular bone spicules, osteoblasts, osteoclasts, blood vessel, and so on can be seen.

From the secondary ossification center to the primary ossification center, the epiphyseal growth plate can be divided into four distinct region in proper order: i.e., the resting zone, the proliferative zone, the hypertrophy and calcified cartilage zone and the ossification zone.

（2）次级骨化中心

随着软骨逐渐生长，在骨两端膨大的软骨中央将会出现次级骨化中心（图3-10），骨组织不断向四周扩大、取代软骨组织，最终只剩关节软骨和骺软骨依然保持软骨状态。次级骨化中心与初级骨化中心结构相似，其内可见不规则的骨小梁、成骨细胞、破骨细胞、血管等。

从次级骨化中心向初级骨化中心骺板可分成4个区，依次是静止区、增生区、肥大钙化区和骨化区。

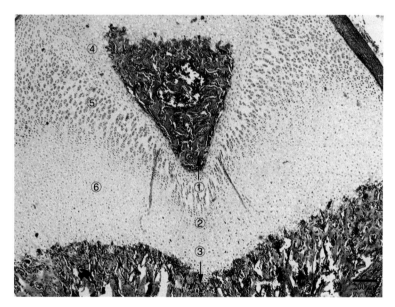

Fig. 3-10　The secondary ossification center, by H.E. stain (demonstration slide)

图3-10　次级骨化中心，HE染色（示教切片）

① secondary ossification center	①次级骨化中心
② epiphyseal plate	②骺板
③ primary ossification center	③初级骨化中心
④ resting zone	④静止区
⑤ proliferative zone	⑤增生区
⑥ hypertrophy and calcified cartilage zone	⑥肥大钙化区
⑦ ossification zone	⑦骨化区

Questions

1.What are the similarities and differences of the bone and the cartilage?

2.How to distinguish the hyaline cartilage, fibrocartilage, dense CT and bone?

3.What is the difference of the perforating fibers and the fibrocartilage?

问题

1.骨和软骨的异同是什么？

2.如何区分透明软骨、纤维软骨、致密结缔组织和骨？

3.穿通纤维和纤维软骨有何区别？

Chapter 4　BLOOD CELLS and HEMOPOIESIS

第四章　血细胞和血细胞发生

Teaching and Learning Objectives

● To identify morphological characteristics of erythrocytes, neutrophils, eosinophils, basophils, monocytes, lymphocytes and platelets in the peripheral blood.

● To identify morphological characteristics of red blood cells at varied stages during erythropoiesis in the bone marrow.

● To identify morphological characteristics of granulocyte at varied stages during granulopoiesis in the bone marrow.

● To identify morphological characteristics of megakaryocytes in the bone marrow.

教学目标

● 辨认血液中红细胞、中性粒细胞、嗜酸性粒细胞、嗜碱性粒细胞、单核细胞、淋巴细胞、血小板的形态特点。

● 辨认骨髓中红系细胞发育过程中的各个阶段的形态特点。

● 辨认骨髓中粒系细胞发育过程中的各个阶段的形态特点。

● 辨认骨髓中的巨核细胞。

1.Blood smear

First, observe the slide under microscope with low power objective and select a field with uniformly dispersed cells. Then, change to the field with a high power objective or to an oil-immersion objective to identify the following cells: erythrocytes, blood platelets and five types of leucocytes (neutrophils, eosinophils, basophils, monocytes and lymphocytes)(Fig. 4-1).

(1) Erythrocytes, 6.5-8.0 μm in diameter, biconcave discoid in shape, anucleate, with homogenous cytoplasm faintly pink in stain, lighter in central than that in peripheral of the cytoplasm.

(2) Blood platelets, 2-4 μm in diameter, usually distributed in cluster, oval in shape, anucleate, with a few blueish-stain granules in the central cytoplasm.

(3) Granulocytes, three types, i.e., neutrophils, eosinophils and basophils, can be distinguished by their "specific" granules, with purplish-blue nuclei.

1.血涂片

先低倍镜下观察涂片，找一个细胞分布比较均匀的视野，再换成高倍镜和油镜观察。需要辨认以下细胞：红细胞、血小板和5种类型的白细胞（中性粒细胞、嗜酸性粒细胞、嗜碱性粒细胞、单核细胞和淋巴细胞）（图4-1）。

（1）红细胞：直径6.5～8.0μm，双凹圆盘状的无核细胞，胞质染成红色，中央较周边染色浅。

（2）血小板：直径2～4μm，常成簇分布。单个血小板呈卵圆形，无核，胞质中央有染成蓝色的颗粒物质。

（3）粒细胞：所有粒细胞核均被染成蓝紫色，根据特殊颗粒的不同染色性，粒细胞可分为3类，即中性粒细胞、嗜酸性粒细胞和嗜碱

1) Neutrophils, 12−15 μm in diameter, account-ed for 50%−70% of the total white blood cells. Their nucleus can be divided into 2−5 lobes joined by thin and poorly visualized strands of chromatin, and their cytoplasm contains numerous fine and poorly visualized granules, as well as azurophilic granules purple in stain.

2) Eosinophils, 12−15 μm in diameter, accounted for 0.5%−3.0% of the total white blood cells. Their nucleus can usually be divided into two lobes connected by a strand of chromatin and their cytoplasm contains numerous eosinophilic granules orange-pink in stain.

3) Basophils, 12−15 μm in diameter, accounted for less than 1% of the total white blood cells, difficult to be found under light microscope. Their nucleus can be divided into 2 to 3 lobes, usually obscured by overlaid specific granules, and their cytoplasm contains numerous basophilic granules of varied sizes and blue-purple in stain.

(4) Agranular leucocytes, no "specific" granules, with azurophilic granules appearing in cytoplasm, finer than those in the granulocytes.

1) Monocytes, 12−20 μm in diameter, accounted for 3%−8% of the total white blood cells, with horse-shoe-or kidney-shaped nucleus and abundant grayish or blueish cytoplasm containing more azurophilic granules.

2) Lymphocytes, 6−18 μm in diameter, accounted for 20%−30% of the total white blood cells in normal adults, small lymphocytes most commonly seen in the blood smear, with round densely-stained nucleus surrounded by a narrow-rim of sky-blue cytoplasm containing purplish azurophilic granules. In medium-sized lymphocytes, their nuclei appear paler and slightly indented in stain, with more abundant cytoplasm containing a few coarse azurophilic granules.

性粒细胞。

1）中性粒细胞：直径12 ~· 15μm，占白细胞的50% ～ 70%。胞核分为2 ～ 5叶，由染色质细丝相连。胞质中含有大量细的难以在光镜下辨认的中性颗粒，也有染成紫色的嗜天青颗粒。

2）嗜酸性粒细胞：直径12 ～ 15μm，占白细胞的0.5% ～ 3.0%。胞核常分为2叶，由染色质细丝相连。胞质中含有大量染成橘红色的嗜酸性颗粒。

3）嗜碱性粒细胞：直径12 ～ 15μm，占白细胞的比例＜1%，故光镜下少见。胞核可分2 ～ 3叶，常被颗粒盖住而无法显示清楚。胞质中含有大量不同大小的染成蓝紫色的嗜碱性颗粒。

（4）无粒细胞：胞质内有嗜天青颗粒，但比粒细胞中颗粒细小，且无特殊颗粒。

1）单核细胞：直径12 ～ 20μm，占白细胞的3% ～ 8%。胞核呈马蹄形或肾形，胞质较多，呈淡灰色或淡蓝色，内含许多紫色的嗜天青颗粒。

2）淋巴细胞：直径6 ～ 18μm，占白细胞的20% ～ 30%。小淋巴细胞最常见，核圆而深染，胞核周有一圈狭窄的天蓝色胞质，内含紫色的嗜天青颗粒。中等大小的淋巴细胞核染色稍浅，有小凹陷，胞质更丰富，内含紫色的嗜天青颗粒。

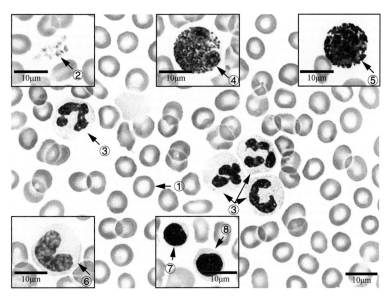

Fig. 4-1　Blood smear, from human, by Wright-Giemsa stain (slide No. C15)

图4-1　血涂片，人，瑞氏-吉姆萨染色（切片No. C15）

①erythrocytes	①红细胞
②blood platelets	②血小板
③neutrophil	③中性粒细胞
④eosinophil	④嗜酸性粒细胞
⑤basophil	⑤嗜碱性粒细胞
⑥monocyte	⑥单核细胞
⑦small lymphocyte	⑦小淋巴细胞
⑧medium-sized lymphocyte	⑧中淋巴细胞

2.Bone marrow smear

First, find a field in the slide with evenly-dispersed and morphologically integrated cells under microscope with low-power objective. Then, observe with a high-power and oil-immersion objectives. It is required to observe morphological characteristics of the cells at varied stages of erythropoiesis and granulopoiesis. When watching a cell in your slide, ask yourself a few questions: "Are there granules in the cell?" If not, it is important to identify "what is the cell and it is in what stage" based on the stain of its nucleus and cytoplasm. If yes, "is there only one kind of granule (azurophilic granule in promyelocyte), or are there two kinds of granules (azurophilic granule and specific granule) ?" If there are both kinds of granules, it is important further to observe nuclear morphology carefully and to identify which cells they are.

(1) Granulopoiesis

1) Myeloblast: round nucleus with lacy chromatin, prominent nucleoli and basophilic cytoplasm of water-color blue in stain without granules.

2.骨髓涂片

先在低倍镜下找一个细胞比较完整且分布均匀的视野，再换成高倍镜和油镜观察。要求观察红系细胞和粒系细胞发育的各个阶段的细胞特点。当看到一个特定细胞时，先考虑几个问题：细胞内是否有颗粒？如果没有颗粒，则要结合核及胞质的染色情况，确定是哪类细胞的哪个阶段；如果有，是一种颗粒（早幼粒细胞中的嗜天青颗粒），还是两种颗粒（嗜天青颗粒和特殊颗粒）都有？如果两种颗粒都有，再观察细胞核的形态，从而最终辨认出是哪种细胞。

（1）粒细胞发生

1）原粒细胞：细胞核染色质稀疏，核仁明显，胞质嗜碱性，染成水彩蓝色，胞质中无颗粒。

2) Promyelocyte: round or oval nucleus with nucleoli possibly seen, basophilic cytoplasm with much azurophilic granules about 0.5 μm in diameter and purplish-red in staining, without specific granules.

3) Myelocyte: with both azurophilic granules and specific granules in cytoplasm, oval and slightly indented nucleus, and more condensed chromatin. Three types of myelocytes can be distinguished based on their chromatophilic properties of the specific granules, i.e., neutrophilic myelocyte, eosinophilic myelocyte and basophilic myelocyte.

Neutrophilic myelocyte: with very small neutrophilic granules in cytoplasm, and not easily resolved under light microscope. As nuclear indentation becomes prominent, it is called neutrophilic metamyelocyte, with horse-shoe-shaped nucleus, and then becoming band-nucleus neutrophilic granulocyte. Subsequently, constriction develops in the two or more places of its nucleus to form lobes connected by delicate strands of chromatin, and the cell is referred to as a mature neutrophilic granulocyte (Fig. 4-2).

2）早幼粒细胞：核圆形或卵圆形，核仁或可见。胞质嗜碱性，胞质中出现许多染成紫红色、直径约0.5μm的嗜天青颗粒，无特殊颗粒。

3）中幼粒细胞：细胞质中既有嗜天青颗粒又有特殊颗粒，胞核卵圆形或有轻微的凹陷，核染色质更加浓缩。根据特殊颗粒嗜色性的不同，分为中性中幼粒细胞、嗜酸性中幼粒细胞和嗜碱性中幼粒细胞。

中性中幼粒细胞：中性颗粒很小，光镜下不易辨认。当胞核凹陷变得明显时，就成为中性晚幼粒细胞，胞核如马蹄形，则成为杆状核的中性粒细胞。随后，胞核的两个到多个部位发生缩窄，形成了由染色质细丝相连的分叶核，就成为成熟的中性粒细胞（图4-2）。

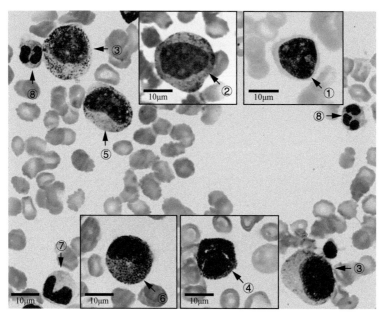

Fig. 4-2　Bone marrow smear, from human, by Wright-Giemsa stain (slide No. C13)
图4-2　骨髓涂片，人，瑞氏－吉姆萨染色（切片No. C13）

①myeloblast	①原粒细胞（成髓细胞）
②promyelocyte	②早幼粒细胞（前髓细胞）
③neutrophilic myelocyte	③中性中幼粒细胞（髓细胞）
④basophilic myelocyte	④嗜碱性中幼粒细胞（髓细胞）
⑤neutrophilic metamyelocyte	⑤中性晚幼粒细胞
⑥eosinophilic metamyelocyte	⑥嗜酸性晚幼粒细胞
⑦band (or stab) cell	⑦杆状核中性粒细胞
⑧mature neutrophil	⑧成熟中性粒细胞

(2) Erythropoiesis

Notice that erythropoiesis (differentiation of red blood cell precursors) is a continuous process, with which one stage grades into the next. Therefore, it is important to decide which stage is at its cell development, based on the changes both in its nucleus and cytoplasm.

1) Proerythroblast: basophilic cytoplasm with oil-painting blue in stain, round nucleus with fine, evenly-distributed and granular chromatin, and prominent nucleoli within the nucleus.

2) Basophilic erythroblast: intensely basophilic cytoplasm without granule, but coarse granular nuclear chromatin without nucleoli.

3) Polychromatophilic erythroblast: cytoplasm grey or alternating pink (acidophilic) and blue (basophilic) in staining, and nucleus with condensed, deeply stained, and coarse heterochromatin appearing a checkerboard pattern (a characteristic alternating dark and light chromatin pattern).

4) Normoblast (orthochromatophilic erythroblast): small, compact, densely stained nucleus, which will soon be extruded, with homogenous eosinophilic cytoplasm red in stain (Fig. 4-3).

（2）红细胞发生

注意：红细胞发生是一个连续的过程，要结合细胞核和胞质的改变来判断一个细胞处于哪个发育阶段。

1）原红细胞：胞质嗜碱性，染成油画蓝色，胞核圆，染色质细颗粒状，稀疏而均匀，核仁明显。

2）早幼红细胞（嗜碱性成红细胞）：胞质强嗜碱性，无颗粒，细胞核染色质粗颗粒状，无核仁。

3）中幼红细胞（嗜多色性成红细胞）：胞质呈灰色或者红蓝相间，染色质浓缩深染，细胞核呈现黑白相间的棋盘状。

4）晚幼红细胞（正成红细胞）：胞核小而固缩，深染，即将排核。胞质嗜酸性，染成均匀的红色（图4-3）。

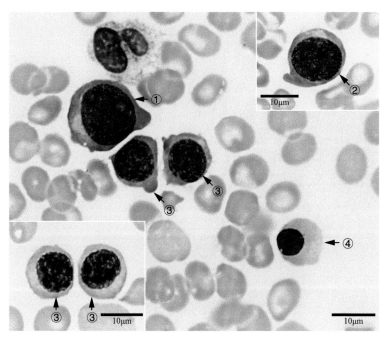

Fig. 4-3　Bone marrow smear, from human, by Wright-Giemsa stain (slide No. C13)

图4-3　骨髓涂片，人，瑞氏-吉姆萨染色（切片 No. C13）

①proerythroblast　　　　　　①原红细胞
②basophilic erythroblast　　　②早幼红细胞
③polychromatophilic　　　　③中幼红细胞
　erythroblast
④orthochromatophilic　　　　④晚幼红细胞
　erythroblast

Reticulocytes: a little bit bigger than mature red blood cell, a blue reticular structure can be seen in cytoplasm, by supravital dyes stain such as brilliant cresyl blue (Fig. 4-4).

网织红细胞：比成熟红细胞略大，使用活体染料煌焦油蓝染色，可见其胞质中有染成蓝色的网状结构（图4-4）。

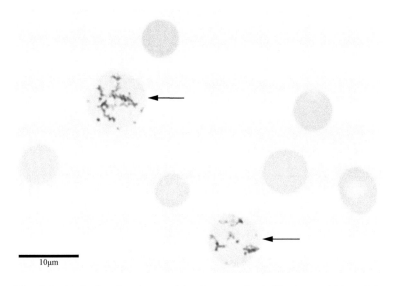

Fig. 4-4　Reticulocytes, human blood smear, by brilliant cresyl blue stain (demonstration slide)

图4-4　网织红细胞，人血涂片，煌焦油蓝染色（示教涂片）

Megakaryocytes: large in size, with large, irregular and multi-lobular nuclei (Fig. 4-5).

巨核细胞：体积大，有大而不规则的多叶核（图4-5）。

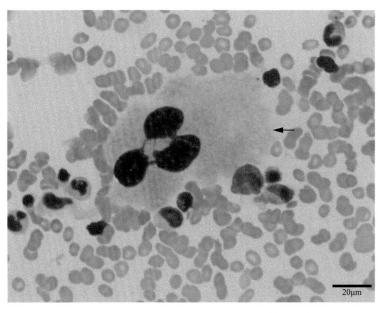

Fig. 4-5　Bone marrow smear, from human, by Wright-Giemsa stain (slide No. C13)

图4-5　骨髓涂片，人，瑞氏-吉姆萨染色（切片No. C13）

Arrow: megakaryocyte　　　　　　　　箭头：巨核细胞

3.Bone marrow

Megakaryocytes, large in size, with multi-lobular nuclei, abundant eosinophilic cytoplasm, and many adipocytes in bone marrow (Fig. 4-6).

3.骨髓切片

巨核细胞体积很大，多叶核，胞质丰富，嗜酸性。骨髓中也有很多脂肪细胞（图4-6）。

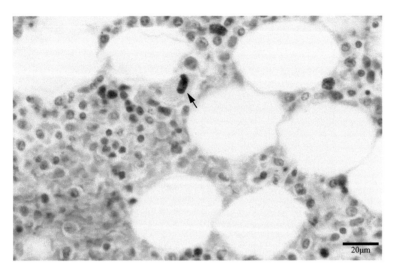

Fig. 4-6   Bone marrow, from human, by H.E. stain (slide No. C14)

图4-6   骨髓切片，人，HE染色（切片No. C14）

Arrow: megakaryocyte   箭头：巨核细胞

Questions

How to distinguish lymphocyte, monocyte from band cell in the light microscope?

问题

如何在光镜下区分淋巴细胞、单核细胞和杆状核中性粒细胞？

Chapter 5   MUSCLE TISSUE
第五章 肌 组 织

Teaching and Learning Objectives

- To identify and describe morphological characteristics of three types of muscle tissue: shape and size of muscle cells (myofibers); number of nuclei per fiber and their location; presence or absence of cross-striation and other specific structures, e.g., intercalated discs, branching of the fibers, etc.
- To identify A band, I band and Z line in the sarcomere.
- To identify perimysium and endomysium in skeletal muscles.
- To distinguish smooth muscle tissue from dense connective tissue.

教学目标

- 辨别并描述3种不同类型肌组织的形态特征：肌细胞（纤维）的形状及大小；细胞核的数量及位置；是否有横纹、闰盘、分支等。
- 辨认肌节明暗带及Z线。
- 辨认骨骼肌的肌束膜及肌内膜。
- 区别平滑肌组织与致密结缔组织。

1.Skeletal muscle

(1) Skeletal muscle

In longitudinal section, skeletal myofiber appears long-cylindrical in shape, with many elongated, oval, nuclei, blunt-round at their two ends, and located just beneath the sarcolemma. Note the difference between nuclei of skeletal muscle fibers and surrounded fibroblasts. Cross-striations with alternating light and dark bands can be seen in the skeletal muscles, where the darker-stained stria is called A band, and lighter-stained stria is called I band in H.E. stain. Cross-striation is clearer by I.H. stain than that by H.E. stain. Dark stained Z line that bisects in the I bands can be seen under oil-immersion objective lens (Fig. 5-1, Fig. 5-2).

1. 骨骼肌

（1）骨骼肌

骨骼肌纵切面上可见骨骼肌纤维呈长圆柱状，细胞核长椭圆形，两端钝圆，多个，位于肌膜下方。请注意骨骼肌细胞核与周围成纤维细胞核的区别。骨骼肌胞质内可见明暗相间的横纹，HE染色切片上深染的为暗带（A band），浅染的为明带（I band）。横纹在铁苏木素染色切片上更为明显。油镜下可见明带中深染的Z线（图5-1，图5-2）。

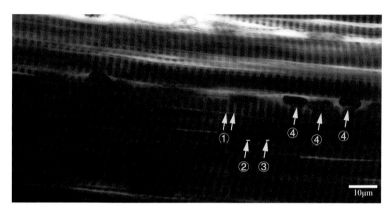

Fig. 5-1　Skeletal muscle, by I.H. stain (slide No. M1)
图5-1　骨骼肌，铁苏木素染色（切片No. M1）

①Z-line (in the middle of I band)　　　　①Z线（明带中央）
②A band　　　　　　　　　　　　　　②暗带
③I band　　　　　　　　　　　　　　③明带
④nuclei of skeletal muscle fiber (or myofiber)　④骨骼肌细胞核

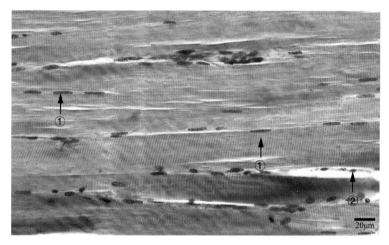

Fig. 5-2　Skeletal muscle, by H.E. stain (slide No. M4)
图5-2　骨骼肌，HE染色（切片No. M4）

①nuclei of skeletal muscle fibers　　　①骨骼肌细胞核
②nucleus of fibroblasts　　　　　　　②成纤维细胞核

(2) Cross-section of skeletal muscles

A whole piece of muscle enclosed by a layer of connective tissue referred to epimysium, can be seen under microscope with low power objective lens. Muscle tissues can be subdivided into several bundles, and each of them is surrounded by connective tissue septum called perimysium. Each single muscle fiber is covered with a delicate sheath of connective tissue, called endomysium. Endomysium, perimysium and epimysium are all continuous in nature. Small blood vessels are present throughout the connective tissue (Fig. 5-3A,

（2）骨骼肌横切面

低倍镜下可见结缔组织包裹整块肌肉，称为肌外膜。肌组织被进一步分成肌束，包绕它们的结缔组织称为肌束膜。每一根肌纤维外纤细的薄层结缔组织称为肌内膜。肌外膜、肌内膜及肌束膜均为连续性的膜。结缔组织中有小血管分布（图5-3A，图5-5）。

Fig. 5-5).

Nuclei of skeletal muscles located peripherally can be clearly seen under microscope with high magnification. Sometimes, cross-section of myofibrils, darkstain cut-ends and regularly arranged in dots can be seen within the cytoplasm (Fig. 5-3B).

高倍镜下明显可见居于周边的骨骼肌细胞核。有时骨骼肌肌浆内可见深染的肌原纤维横断面，点状整齐排列（图5-3B）。

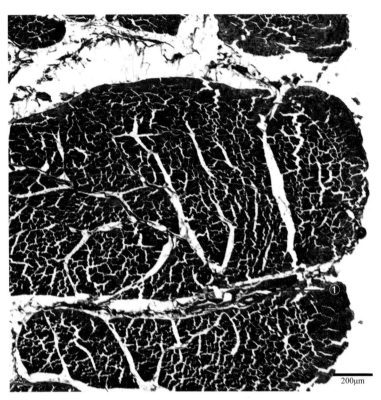

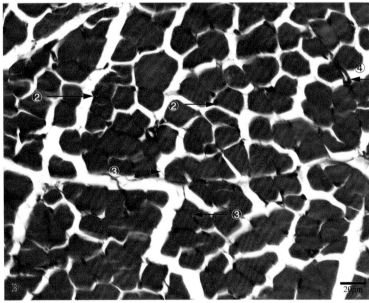

Fig. 5-3 Cross-section of skeletal muscle, by H.E. stain (slide No. M2)

图5-3 骨骼肌，横切，HE染色（切片No. M2）

A.Low-power objective;	A. 低倍镜；
B.High-Power objective	B. 高倍镜
①perimysium	①肌束膜
②nuclei of skeletal muscle fibers	②骨骼肌细胞核
③endomysium	③肌内膜
④blood vessel	④血管

(3) Tongue

Skeletal muscle fibers of longitudinal, transverse or oblique sections interwoven together can be been in the section, with such muscular orientation allowing mobility of tongue towards varied directions. Connective tissue between small fascicle of muscle penetrating into lamina propria, makes its mucous membrane strongly adherent to muscular core, with small salivary glands among it (Fig. 5-4).

（3）舌

舌切片上可见纵切、横切或斜切的骨骼肌纤维交织排列。舌中各个方向走行的肌纤维使得舌可在各方向运动。肌束间的结缔组织与舌黏膜固有层相延续，因此可以将黏膜固定在骨骼肌核心上。这些结缔组织间有小唾液腺分布（图5-4）。

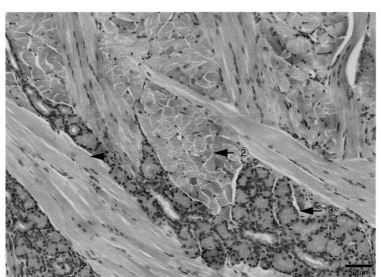

Fig. 5-4   Tongue, by H.E. stain (slide No. DT2)

图5-4　舌，HE染色（切片No. DT2）

①longitudinal section of skeletal muscle fibers	①骨骼肌纤维纵切
②cross-section of skeletal muscle fibers	②骨骼肌纤维横切
③small salivary gland	③小唾液腺

A section of extrinsic eye muscle from rabbit after injecting Indian ink via its ophthalmic artery, show blood vessels and their branches in dark stain among skeletal muscle fibers（Fig.5-5）.

兔眼动脉注射印度墨汁后的眼外肌切片，可见血管及其分支显示为黑色分支状，走行于骨骼肌纤维之间（图5-5）。

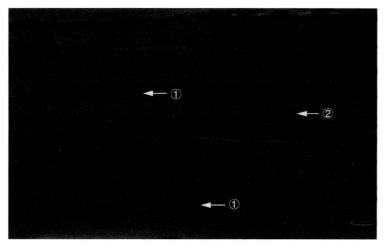

Fig. 5-5   Extrinsic eye muscle, from rabbit, by Indian ink injection (demonstration slide)

图5-5　兔眼肌，印度墨汁注射（示教切片）

①capillary	①毛细血管
②skeletal muscle fiber	②骨骼肌纤维

2.Cardiac muscle (Myocardium)

Under low power objective, muscle fibers are arranged in bundles, with centrally-located nuclei, sometimes binucleate. Different orientations of these fiber bundles can be seen in the section (Fig. 5-6). Under high power objective, cross-striation can be seen in longitudinal section of cardiac muscle fibers, but not so apparent as that seen in skeletal muscle. Cardiac muscle fibers branch and anastomose mutually to form network. Note that the intercalated discs can be seen in longitudinally oriented bundles, appearing dark-stained at Z line level, vertical to long axis of cardiac muscle fibers and showing a thread or steplike profile. Centrally located nucleus, or some light stain juxtanuclear region, if nucleus is not included in the section, can be seen in cross-section of cardiac muscle. Yellowish-brown pigment (i.e., lipofuscin) granules can be seen in some juxtanuclear region (Fig. 5-7).

2.心肌（心肌膜）

低倍镜下，肌纤维排列成束，心肌纤维细胞核居中，有时可见双核，切面上可见不同走向的纤维（图5-6）。高倍镜下，纵切心肌纤维可见横纹，但不如骨骼肌明显。心肌纤维有分支，相互吻合成网状。注意：在纵切面上可以见到闰盘，在Z线水平，深染，并与心肌纤维长轴垂直，呈线状或阶梯状。横切心肌纤维可见细胞核居中，如未切到核可见浅染的核周区，有些核周区可见棕黄色脂褐素颗粒（图5-7）。

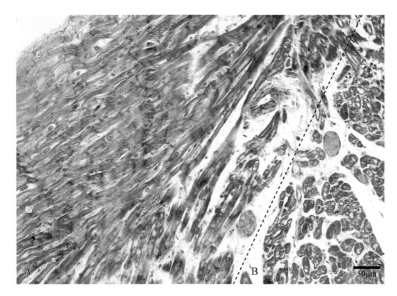

Fig. 5-6　Cardiac muscle, by H.E. stain (slide No. M3)
图5-6　心肌，HE染色（切片No. M3）

A.Longitudinal section of cardiac muscle;　　A.心肌纵切；

B.Cross-section of cardiac muscle　　　　　B.心肌横切

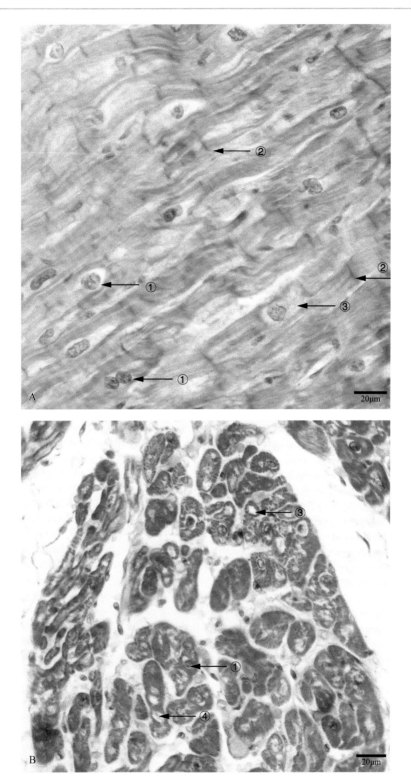

Fig. 5-7　Cardiac muscle, by H.E. stain (slide No. M3)

图 5-7　心肌，HE 染色（切片 No. M3）

A.Longitudinal section; B.Cross section　　A.纵切片；B.横切片

①nuclei of cardiac muscle　　　　　　　①心肌细胞核

②intercalated disc　　　　　　　　　　　②闰盘

③juxtanuclear region　　　　　　　　　　③核周区

④lipofuscin pigment　　　　　　　　　　④脂褐素

3.Smooth muscle

(1) Urinary bladder

Cells of bundles of smooth muscles oriented from varied planes can be observed under microscope with low magnification, surrounded and demarcated by collagenous fibers. Observe morphological characteristics of smooth muscle cells at its longitudinal section: elongate spindle-shaped cells, single-nucleate in cigar-shape, nucleus centrally located along its longitudinal axis in parallel with that of smooth muscle cells, and with no cross-striation in its cytoplasm. Varied sizes of smooth muscle can be seen in cross-sections, but centrally-located nucleus can just be seen in some cross-sections, that's because only mid-portion of spindle-shaped cells are occupied by nucleus. It is usually difficult to distinguish smooth muscle from fibrous connective tissue scattered in the slide by H.E. stain, due to cytoplasm of both smooth muscle cells and collagenous fibers appearing acidophilic. Nuclei of fibroblasts are smaller and densely stained, however, nuclei of smooth muscles appear elongate and round, with two to three times in length as those of fibroblasts, with lightly-stained loose chromatin (Fig. 5-8).

3.平滑肌

（1）膀胱

低倍镜下可见膀胱壁上不同走向的平滑肌细胞束，成束的平滑肌细胞周围有胶原纤维包绕。在纵切面观察平滑肌细胞形态，梭形、单个核，呈雪茄烟状，居中，长轴与平滑肌细胞长轴一致，胞质内没有横纹。平滑肌横切面上可见不同大小的切面，由于细胞核只占据整个梭形细胞的中间部位，因此只有部分细胞横切面能看到居中的细胞核。胶原纤维和平滑肌胞质均呈嗜酸性，因此在HE染色的切片上，通常比较难以区分散在结缔组织中的平滑肌细胞。成纤维细胞的核小而深染，而平滑肌核长圆，染色质疏松，长度可以是成纤维细胞核的2～3倍（图5-8）。

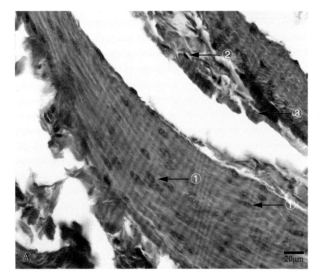 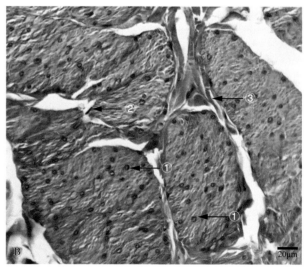

Fig. 5-8　Smooth muscle, urinary bladder, by H.E. stain (slide No. Ur3)
图5-8　平滑肌，膀胱，HE染色（切片No. Ur3）

A.smooth muscle fibers in longitudinal section; B.Smooth muscle fibers in cross-section

①nuclei of smooth muscle
②nucleus of fibroblast
③collagenous fibers

A.纵切平滑肌；B.横切平滑肌

①平滑肌细胞核
②成纤维细胞核
③胶原纤维

(2) Scalp

Epithelium, hair follicles and dermis composed of connective tissue can be seen under microscope with low magnification. Hair follicles formed in the continuous from epidermis to dermis can be found. Arrector pili muscles composed of a bundle of smooth muscles near hair follicles can be identified in longitudinal, cross-sectional or oblique sections. Note to distinguish the lightly-stained nuclei of smooth muscle cells from the densely-stained nuclei of fibroblasts (Fig. 5-9).

（2）头皮

低倍镜下观察切片，可见表皮、毛囊以及结缔组织构成的真皮。找到表皮向真皮方向延续形成的毛囊，毛囊附近可见一束平滑肌构成的立毛肌，可纵切、横切或斜切。注意区分浅染的平滑肌细胞核与深染的成纤维细胞核（图5-9）。

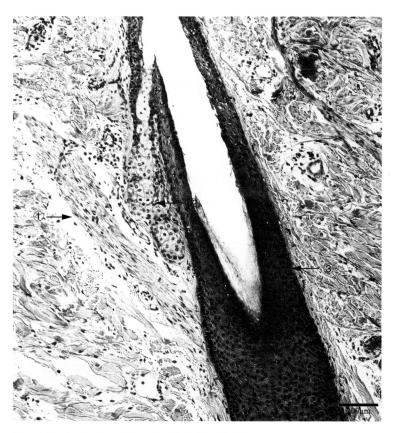

Fig. 5-9　Scalp, by H.E. stain (slide No. Sk3)
图5-9　头皮，HE染色（切片No. Sk3）

①arrector pili muscle　　　　①立毛肌
②sebaceous gland　　　　　②皮脂腺
③hair follicle　　　　　　　③毛囊

Smooth muscle cells scatter among acini of the prostate. Observe single, spindle-shaped cell with elongate, round nucleus and eosinophilic cytoplasm (Fig. 5-10).

前列腺中平滑肌细胞散在分布于腺泡之间。观察单个细胞的梭形形态，长圆的细胞核以及嗜酸性胞质（图5-10）。

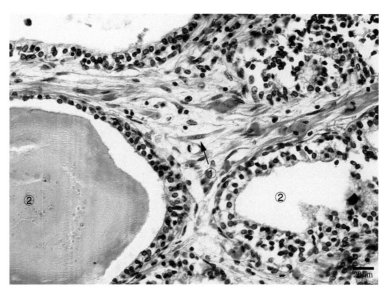

Fig. 5-10　Scattered smooth muscle cells, prostate, by H.E. stain (demonstration slide)

图5-10　散在的平滑肌细胞，前列腺，HE染色（示教切片）

①smooth muscle cell　　　　　　　①平滑肌细胞
②prostate acini　　　　　　　　　②前列腺腺泡

Questions

1.Fill out the following form after observation.

	Skeletal muscle	Cardiac muscle	Smooth muscle
location			
morphology			
shape			
striation			
nucleus			
myofibrils			
T-tubules			
sarcoplasmic reticulum			
cell-cell junctions			
other components			
function			
type of innervation			
type of contraction			
growth and regeneration			
mitosis			
regeneration			

2.Try to describe the difference between smooth muscle and dense connective tissue.

问题

1. 观察后填表。

	骨骼肌	心肌	平滑肌
分布部位			
形态学			
形状			
横纹			
核			
肌纤维			
T-小管			
肌浆网			
细胞间连接			
其他（结构）成分			
功能			
神经分布（支配）类型			
收缩类型			
生长和再生			
有丝分裂			
再生			

2. 试描述平滑肌与致密结缔组织的区别。

Chapter 6 NERVE TISSUE

第六章 神经组织

Teaching and Learning Objectives

- To identify neurons in H.E. stain and neurofibrils and synapses button in silver stain.
- To identify four types of neuroglia in central nervous system in H.E. stain and special (silver) stain.
- To identify peripheral nerves and Schwann cells and distinguish myelinated nerve fibers from unmyelinated ones.
- To identify free nerve endings and encapsulated nerve endings.
- To identify spinal ganglia and sympathetic ganglia.

教学目标

- HE染色下辨认神经元，特殊染色下辨认神经原纤维、突触扣结。
- HE染色及特殊染色下辨认中枢神经系统中4种类型胶质细胞。
- 辨认外周神经和施万细胞，区分有髓和无髓神经纤维。
- 辨认游离神经末梢和有被囊的神经末梢。
- 辨认脊神经节和交感神经节。

1.Neurons

(1) Spinal cord, by H.E. stain

In cross-section of spinal cord, nerve cells (neurons) are clustered in the central gray matter appearing in H shape, and nerve fibers are mainly located in the peripheral white matter. Neurons have large cell bodies, round and large "hawk-eye" nuclei with loose chromatin, prominent nucleolus and abundant cytoplasm containing much basophilic granules called Nissl bodies, a characteristic structure of neuron (Fig. 6-1). Nissl bodies can extend into the proximal dendrites, but are absent in the axons extending from axon-hillock (Fig. 6-2).

1.神经元

（1）脊髓，HE染色

脊髓横切面上，神经元胞体位于中央的H型灰质，而神经纤维主要位于外周白质。神经元胞体体积大，胞核大而圆，染色质疏松，核仁明显，呈"鹰眼"状；胞质丰富，含较多嗜碱性斑块，称尼氏体，是神经元特征性结构（图6-1）。尼氏体可以出现在树突，而轴突从轴丘起，无尼氏体（图6-2）。

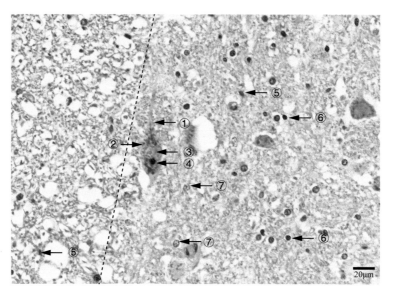

Fig. 6-1　Spinal cord, by H.E. stain (slide No. N1)

图6-1　脊髓，HE染色（切片No. N1）

Left: white matter; Right: gray matter　　　　左侧：白质；右侧：灰质

①dendrite　　　　　　　　　　　　　　　①神经元树突

②Nissl bodies　　　　　　　　　　　　　②尼氏体

③nuclear membrane　　　　　　　　　　③核膜

④nucleolus　　　　　　　　　　　　　　④核仁

⑤microglia　　　　　　　　　　　　　　⑤小胶质细胞

⑥oligodendrocytes　　　　　　　　　　　⑥少突胶质细胞

⑦astrocytes　　　　　　　　　　　　　　⑦星形胶质细胞

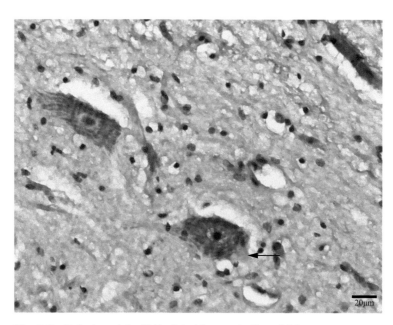

Fig. 6-2　Spinal cord, by H.E. stain (demonstration slide)

图6-2　脊髓，HE染色（示教切片）

Arrow: axon-hillock　　　　　　　　　　箭头：轴丘

(2) Neurons, Cajal's silver stain

In one demonstration slide of rabbit brain with Cajal's sliver stain, yellowish-brown motor neurons can be seen with dark thinner filaments in their cytoplasm and processes, i.e., neurofibrils, forming an important cellular skeletal element of them (Fig. 6-3).

In another demonstration slide of spinal cord with silver stain, synapses appear as dark "comma"-like dots, called synapses buttons, along the cell membranes of neuron somas and processes (Fig. 6-4).

（2）神经元，卡哈尔银染

示教切片［兔脑，卡哈尔（Cajal）银染］中，可见棕黄色运动神经元，胞质及突起中均有黑色细丝，即神经原纤维，为神经元中重要细胞骨架成分（图6-3）。

另一示教切片银染的脊髓中，突触呈黑色蝌蚪样，又称突触扣结，可见于神经元胞体及突起的细胞膜上（图6-4）。

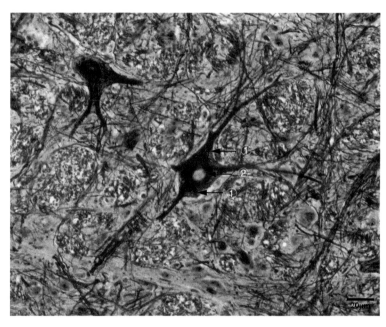

Fig. 6-3　Rabbit brain, by Cajal sliver stain (demonstration slide)

图6-3　兔脑，卡哈尔银染（示教切片）

①neurofibrils　　　　　　①神经原纤维
②unstained nucleus of　　②未着色的神经元细
　　neuron　　　　　　　　胞核

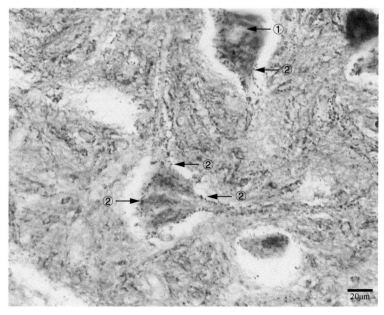

Fig. 6-4　Spinal cord from cat, by Cajal stain (demonstration slide)

图6-4　猫脊髓，卡哈尔染色（示教切片）

①unstained nucleus of　　①未着色的神经元细
　　neuron　　　　　　　　胞核
②synapse button　　　　　②突触扣结

2.Neuroglial cells

(1) Spinal cord, by H.E. stain

Prominent cytoplasm can be seen in neurons of spinal gray matter with H.E. stain. However, perinuclear cytoplasm and process of neuroglial cells cannot easily be identified. Varied types of neuroglial cells can be identified according to their nucleus' morphological characteristics. Astrocyte is one of the largest neuroglia cells, with larger, round and pale-stain nucleus, but nucleus of oligodendrocyte is round, smaller and darker-stain. That with the smallest and irregular nucleus is microglia (Fig. 6-1). Ependymal cells line around the central canal of spinal cord, as columnar or cuboidal epithelia (Fig. 6-5).

2.神经胶质细胞

（1）脊髓，HE染色

HE染色中，灰质中的神经元可以看到明显的胞质，而胶质细胞胞质和突起均不易辨认。可以通过细胞核形态特征辨认不同类型胶质细胞，星形胶质细胞是最大的胶质细胞，胞核较大，圆，浅染；少突胶质细胞核圆形，小而深染；最小且形状不规则的细胞核属于小胶质细胞（图6-1）。室管膜细胞贴附于脊髓中央管，为柱状或立方形上皮样细胞（图6-5）。

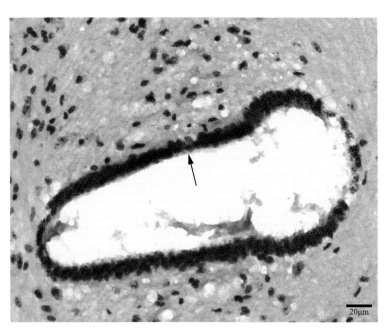

Fig. 6-5　Central cannal of spinal cord, by H.E. stain (demonstration slide)
图6-5　脊髓中央管，HE染色（示教切片）

Arrow: ependymal cells　　　　　　　　箭头：室管膜细胞

(2) Cerebrum, by Golgi stain

In the thick slide of cerebrum, cell bodies and processes of neurons and neuroglial cells are black in Golgi stain, and so can easily be identified. The bodies of cerebral pyramidal cells appear large and triangular in shape, with elongate and less processes. Protoplasmic astrocytes present mainly in the gray matter, with smaller bodies, and shorter, more branched processes. Fibrous astrocytes present mainly in the white matter, with long and less-branched processes, sometimes with the process ends attaching to the capillary walls (Fig. 6-6). The processes of oligodendrocytes may not easily be stained, so only unstained nucleus can be seen in the densely-stained cell bodies (Fig. 6-7). microglia can be identified in special stain (Fig. 6-8, rabbit brain, demonstration slide).

（2）大脑，高尔基染色

在大脑厚片高尔基染色中，神经元和神经胶质细胞的胞体及其突起均能被染为黑色，从而易于辨识。大脑锥体细胞胞体大，呈三角形，突起长而少。原浆型星形胶质细胞主要分布于灰质，胞体小而突起多，短，呈分支状。纤维型星形胶质细胞主要分布于白质，突起长而分支少，有时可见突起形成脚板样黏附于毛细血管（图6-6）。少突胶质细胞突起不易染色，因此仅能见深染胞体中有不着色的细胞核，突起极少（图6-7）。小胶质细胞经特殊染色可分辨（图6-8，示教兔脑）。

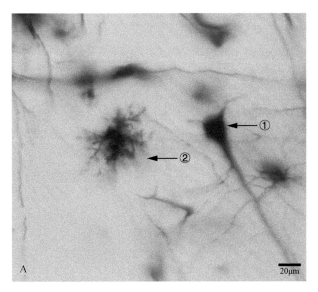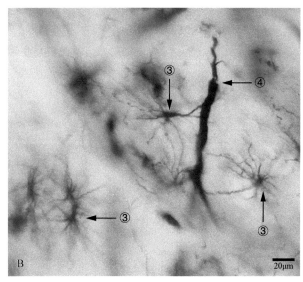

Fig. 6-6   Cerebrum, from cat, by Golgi stain (slide No. N3)
图6-6   猫大脑，高尔基染色（切片No. N3）

A. Gray matter; B. White matter
① neuron
② protoplasmic astrocytes
③ fibrous astrocytes
④ blood vessel

A. 灰质；B. 白质
① 神经元
② 原浆型星形胶质细胞
③ 纤维型星形胶质细胞
④ 血管

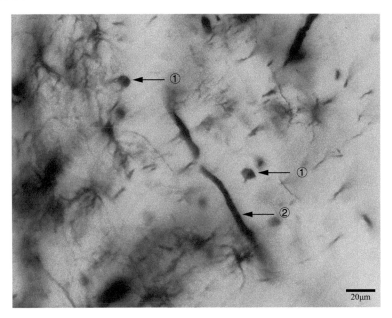

Fig. 6-7   Cerebrum, by Golgi stain (demonstration slide)
图6-7   猫大脑，高尔基染色（示教切片）

① oligodendrocyte   ①少突胶质细胞
② blood vessel   ②血管

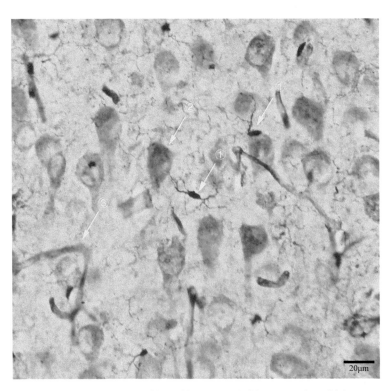

Fig. 6-8   Cerebrum, from rabbit, by Hortega stain (demonstration slide)
图6-8   小兔大脑，Hortega镀银染色（示教切片）

① microglia cell   ①小胶质细胞
② neuron   ②神经元
③ blood vessel   ③血管

3.Nerve Fiber

Nerve fiber is referred to axon of neuron, usually clustered in bundles containing several to over a million fibers. Bundles of nerve fibers are called peripheral nerves in peripheral nervous system (PNS), and transmission fascicles (or nerve fiber tract) in central nervous system (CNS). Peripheral nerves consist of three major elements: axons, Schwann cells (may forming myelin sheath around axon) and connective tissue including blood vessels served as supporting roles.

(1) Sciatic nerve, from human, by H.E. stain

In cross-section of human sciatic nerve, both epineurium and perineurium can be seen under microscope with low-power objective. Epineurium is composed of dense connective tissue, surrounding the whole piece of nerve. While perineurium is composed of connective tissue too, with several layers of pink stained flat fibroblasts served as insulation to help recognize nerve bundle in the other organs. With high-power objective lens, the axons are pink dots surrounded by pale stain myelin sheath. Lots of lipid in the membrane of Schwann cells forming myelin sheath have been removed by organic solvents in preparation of the paraffin slide, so myelin sheaths are stained light. Nuclei of Schwann cells usually adhere to the edge of myelin sheaths, presenting semi-oval in shape and light stain, with loose chromatin. Thin pink stained collagenous fiber around a piece of outer myelin nerve fiber can be seen and is called endoneurium (Fig. 6-9).

3.神经纤维

神经纤维是指神经元轴突，通常集结成束状，数量从几根到几百万根不等，在周围神经系统中被称为外周神经，在中枢神经系统中被称为传导束。外周神经中含有3种主要成分：轴突、施万细胞（可形成围绕轴突的髓鞘）以及起到支持作用的结缔组织，包括血管。

（1）人坐骨神经，HE染色

在低倍镜下观察，人坐骨神经横切，可见神经外膜及神经束膜：神经外膜包绕整根神经外周，为致密结缔组织；神经束膜也是结缔组织，但其中含有数层粉染的扁平成纤维细胞，形成神经束膜上皮，起到绝缘作用，同时也能帮助我们在其他器官中辨认神经束。高倍镜下观察有髓神经纤维，中央的轴突呈粉红点状，周围浅染的部位为髓鞘，构成髓鞘的施万细胞膜中大量的脂质在蜡片制作过程中被有机溶剂去除而呈不着色状态。施万细胞核常贴附于髓鞘边缘，半椭圆形，核染色质疏松。一根有髓神经纤维的外沿可见粉染的细胶原纤维，为神经内膜（图6-9）。

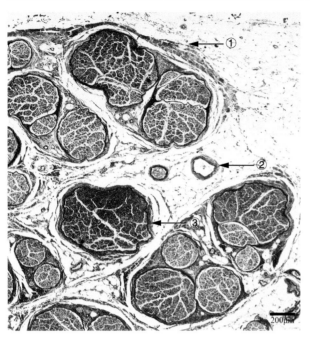
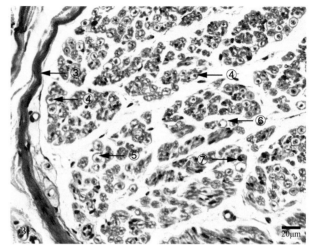

Fig. 6-9　Sciatic nerve, from human, by H.E. stain (slide No. N6)

图6-9　人坐骨神经，HE染色（切片No. N6）

A. Under low power objective; B. Under high power objective

A. 低倍镜；B. 高倍镜

①epineurium

②blood vessel

③perineurium

④axon

⑤myelin sheath

⑥endoneurium

⑦nucleus of Schwann cell

①神经外膜

②血管

③神经束膜

④轴突

⑤髓鞘

⑥神经内膜

⑦施万细胞核

(2) Sciatic nerve, from cat, by H.E. stain

This slide contains both longitudinal section and cross-section of cat sciatic nerve. In longitudinal section, the axons appear as a pink thread-like matter surrounded by pale-stain myelin sheath, and the node of Ranvier is quite prominent, with pink-stain collagenous fibers around it, called endoneurium (Fig. 6-10).

（2）猫坐骨神经，HE染色

切片显示了猫坐骨神经纵切与横切。在纵切面上，轴突显示为粉色线状，周围包绕浅色髓鞘，可见明显的郎飞结，周围粉染的胶原纤维为神经内膜（图6-10）。

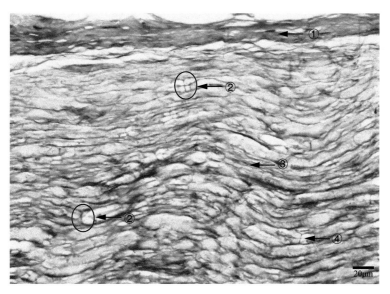

Fig. 6-10　Sciatic nerve, from cat, by H.E. stain (slide No. N7)
图6-10　猫坐骨神经，HE染色（切片No. N7）

①perineurium	①神经束膜
②node of Ranvier	②郎飞结
③nucleus of Schwann cell	③施万细胞核
④axon	④轴突

(3) Sciatic nerve, by osmic acid stain

Myelin sheath is preserved in this specific preparation and presents as black in color by osmic acid (osmium tetroxide) stain. Relationship between myelin sheath and axon can be seen in both longitudinal section and cross-section of sciatic nerve. Also, the nodes of Ranvier can be apparently observed in longitudinal section (Fig. 6-11).

（3）坐骨神经，铌酸染色

特殊制片保留髓鞘，铌酸染色使髓鞘呈黑色，可在横切及纵切面观察髓鞘与轴突关系，也可在纵切面上观察到明显的郎飞结（图6-11）。

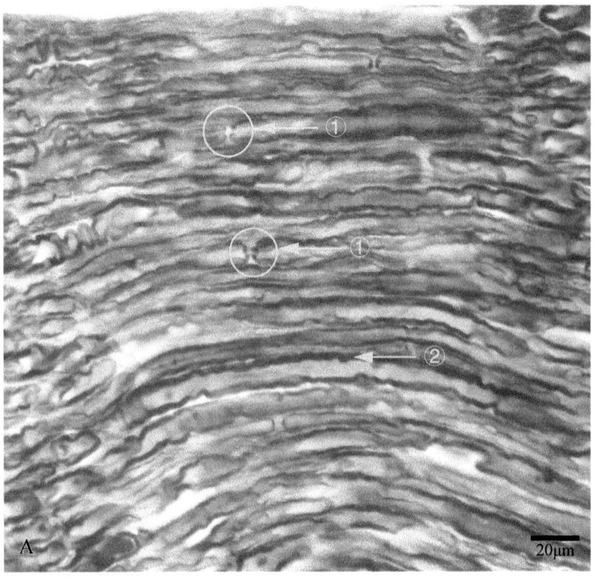

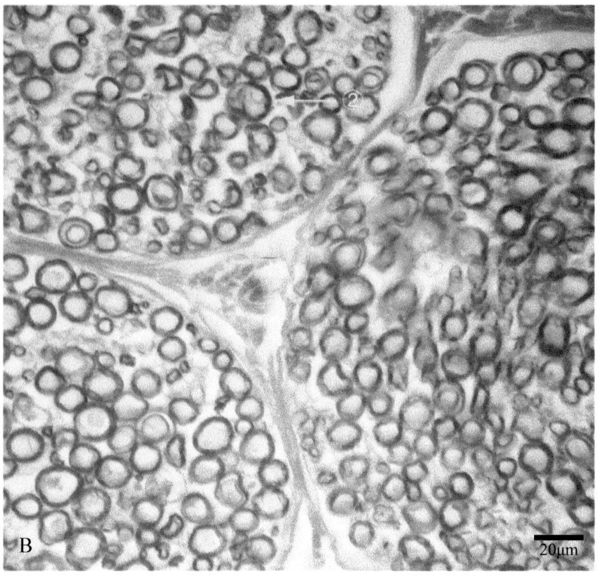

Fig. 6-11 Sciatic nerve, by osmic acid stain (slide No. N8)
图6-11 坐骨神经，锇酸染色（切片No. N8）

A. Longitudinal section; B. Cross section
①node of Ranvier
②myelin sheath

A. 纵切片；B. 横切片
①郎飞结
②髓鞘

(4) Sciatic nerve, from rabbit, by Mallory trichrome stain

Cytoplasm and collagenous fiber can be stained as blue, myelin sheath protein as yellowish-orange, and nucleus as purplish-red by Mallory trichrome stain, and blueish-gray axon surrounded by orange myelin sheath can be seen, with elongated, purplish-red nucleus of the Schwann cells. All epineurium, perineurium and endoneurium surround neurofiber containing collagen fibers presenting blue in varied degrees and can be easily distinguished in both longitudinal and cross sections of sciatic nerve (Fig. 6-12).

（4）兔坐骨神经，马洛里三色染色

马洛里三色染色后细胞质及胶原纤维呈蓝色，髓鞘蛋白呈橘黄色，细胞核呈紫红色。切片上可见灰蓝色的轴突包绕有橘黄色的髓鞘，边缘有长椭圆形紫红色的施万细胞核。神经纤维周围的神经内膜、神经束膜和神经外膜都含有胶原纤维成分而呈不同深浅的蓝色，易于辨认（图6-12）。

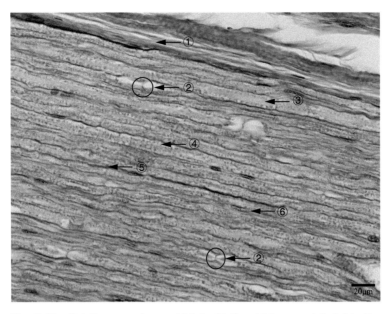

Fig. 6-12　Sciatic nerve, from rabbit, by Mallory trichrome stain (slide No. N9)

图6-12　兔坐骨神经，Mallory三色染色（切片No. N9）

①perineurium	①神经束膜
②node of Ranvier	②郎飞结
③axon	③轴突
④myelin sheath	④髓鞘
⑤endoneurium	⑤神经内膜
⑥nucleus of Schwann cell	⑥施万细胞核

(5) Sympathetic nerve, from human, by I.H. stain

Sympathetic nerve contains lots of unmyelinated fibers and a few of myelinated fibers. Unmyelinated fibers present undulant in shape, evenly-stained, and containing more nuclei of Schwann cells. Axon of myelinated fibers is surrounded by pale-stain myelin sheath structure, and sometimes Schmidt-Lanterman clefts like fish-bone can be seen in myelin sheath (Fig. 6-13).

（5）人交感神经，铁苏木素染色

交感神经含有较多的无髓神经纤维和少量有髓神经纤维。无髓神经纤维呈波浪状，染色均匀，含较多的施万细胞核。有髓神经纤维轴突周围有浅淡的髓鞘结构，有时髓鞘中可见鱼骨刺样的施－兰切迹（图6-13）。

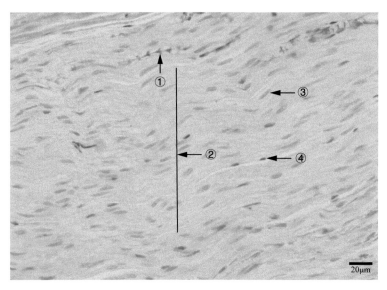

Fig. 6-13　Sympathetic nerve, from human, by I.H. stain (slide No. N10)
图6-13　人交感神经，铁苏木素染色（切片No. N10）

①Schmidt-Lanterman cleft　　　①施－兰切迹
②unmyelinated nerve fiber　　　②无髓神经纤维
③nucleus of Schwann cell　　　③施万细胞核
④nucleus of fibroblast　　　　④成纤维细胞核

4.Nerve Endings

(1) Finger skin, from human, by H.E. stain

Two types of encapsulated sensory nerve endings can be seen in section of finger skin, i.e., Meissner's (or tactile) corpuscle and Pacinian (or lamellar) corpuscle. Meissner's corpuscle presents short-rod in shape, and is located beneath the stratified squamous epithelium and at the superficial layer of dermis, with Schwann cells arranged in parallel. Sensory nerve endings wind among Schwann cells and cannot be identified in H.E. stain, but can be done in silver stain (demonstration slide). Pacinian corpuscle is located at the deeper dermis, with demyelinated nerve ending at the center and surrounded by collagenous fibers and Schwann cells arranged in elliptical structure in the section, just resembling sliced onion (Fig. 6-14, Fig. 6-15).

4.神经末梢

（1）指皮，人，HE染色

指皮切片中可见两种有被囊的感觉神经末梢：触觉小体和环层小体。触觉小体位于复层扁平上皮下方，真皮的浅层，呈短棒状，施万细胞平行排列，感觉神经纤维末梢螺旋走形于施万细胞间，HE染色上不能辨认神经末梢，但银染可显示（示教切片）。环层小体位于真皮深部，中央是脱髓鞘的神经末梢，周围环绕同心圆状排列的胶原纤维及施万细胞，切面呈洋葱片样（图6-14，图6-15）。

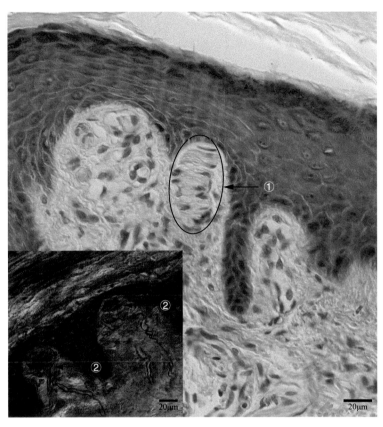

Fig. 6-14　Finger skin, from human, by H.E. stain (slide No. Sk1)
Inserted (demonstration slide) : by Cajal stain
图6-14　指皮，人，HE染色（切片 No. Sk1.），图中图（示教切片）：卡哈尔染色

①meissner corpuscle　　　　　　①触觉小体
②nerve fibers　　　　　　　　　②神经纤维

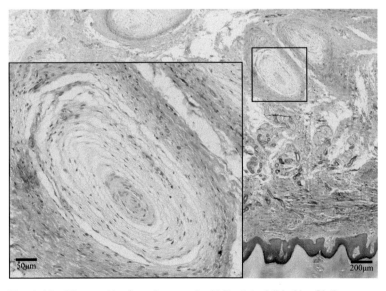

Fig. 6-15　Finger skin, from human, by H.E. stain (slide No. Sk1)
图6-15　指皮，人，HE染色（切片 No. Sk1）

Pacinian corpuscle　　　　　　　环层小体

Free nerve ending was stained as black thread extending between keratinocytes of epidermis and around hair follisles by silver stain (Fig. 6-16).

游离神经末梢银染呈黑色细线状，可见其伸入上皮细胞间及毛囊周围（图6-16）。

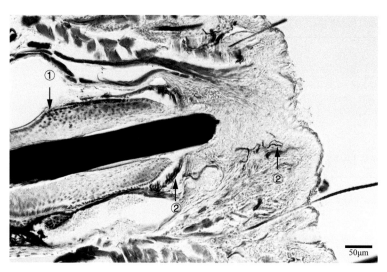

Fig. 6-16　Rat vibrissa, by Gros-Bielchowsky stain (demonstration slide)

图6-16　大鼠触须，Gros-Bielchowsky染色（示教切片）

①vibrissa hair follicle
②nerve ending

①触须毛囊
②神经末梢

(2) Motor end plate and muscle spindle

Myofibers present dark purple, while nerve fibers and their endings present black in the slide of skeletal muscle torn into tiny pieces and stained by gold chloride method. The ends of motor nerve fibers branch and adhere to the surface of skeletal muscle fibers forming motor end plates. The fusiform structure of muscle as a whole appears spindle in shape among muscle fibers. Intrafusal myofibril is trapped by thin capsule, which is thinner than extrafusal one, with cross-striation and centrally-located nucleus (Fig. 6-17).

（2）运动终板与肌梭

骨骼肌撕片氯化金染色中，肌纤维呈深紫色，神经纤维及末梢呈黑色。运动神经纤维末端分支，贴附于骨骼肌纤维表面形成运动终板。肌梭整体呈梭形，位于肌纤维之间。HE染色中可见梭内肌纤维有被囊包裹，梭内肌纤维较梭外肌纤维细，有横纹，细胞核居中（图6-17）。

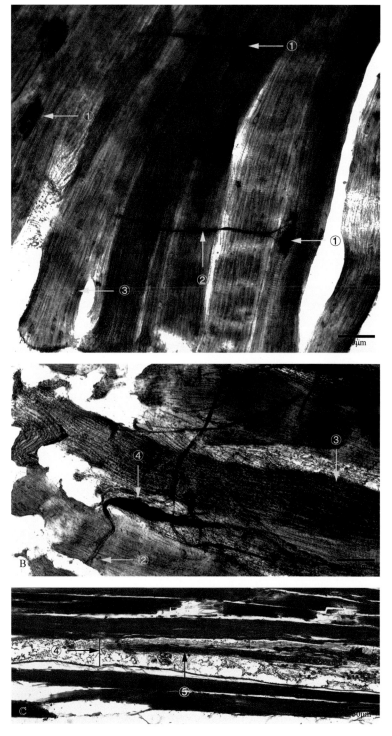

Fig. 6-17　Motor end plate and muscle spindle (demonstration slide)
图6-17　运动终板与肌梭（示教切片）

A, B: Skeletal muscle torn into tiny pieces, by gold chloride stain; C: Skeletal muscle by H.E. stain

①motor end plate
②nerve fiber
③skeletal muscle fiber
④muscle spindle
⑤intrafusal myofibril

A，B：骨骼肌撕片，氯化金染色；C：骨骼肌，HE染色

①运动终板
②神经纤维
③骨骼肌纤维
④肌梭
⑤梭内肌纤维

5.Ganglion

The structure with cluster of neuron bodies, outside of the central nervous system, is called ganglion.

(1) Spinal ganglia (dorsal root ganglia), by H.E. stain

The outermost layer of ganglion is surrounded by dense connective tissue capsule, within which neurons distribute in groups and are separated by fascicles of nerve fibers. Spinal ganglia contain pseudo-unipolar neurons, but cannot be identified in this slide. Their cell bodies are surrounded by satellite cells with small and round nuclei (Fig. 6-18).

5.神经节

中枢神经系统以外的神经元胞体聚集的结构称为神经节。

（1）脊神经节（背根神经节），HE染色

神经节最外包绕一层结缔组织被膜，内有成群分布的神经元，之间走行有神经纤维束。脊神经节含有假单极神经元，但在切片上无法分辨，其胞体周围包绕有小、圆核的卫星细胞（图6-18）。

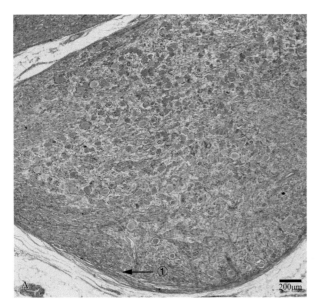
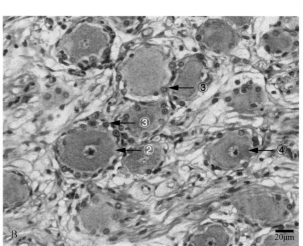

Fig. 6-18　Spinal ganglia (dorsal root ganglia) , by H.E. stain (slide No. N11)
图6-18　脊神经节（背根神经节），HE染色（切片No. N11）

A.Under Low power objective; B.Under high power objective
①capsule
②neuron
③satellite cell
④lipofuscin pigment

A.低倍镜；B.高倍镜
①被膜
②神经元
③卫星细胞
④脂褐素

(2) Cervical sympathetic ganglia, by H.E. stain

Neuron bodies in sympathetic ganglia are smaller than those in spinal ganglia, scattered in distribution, with eccentric nuclei, less satellite cells and more unmyelinated fibers (Fig. 6-19).

（2）颈交感神经节，HE染色

交感神经节中神经元胞体较小，散在分布，胞核常偏心，卫星细胞数量少，无髓神经纤维较多（图6-19）。

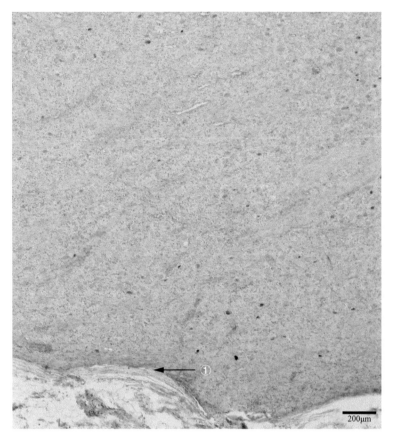

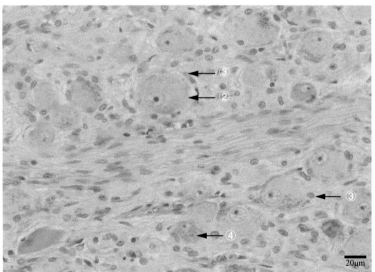

Fig. 6-19   Cervical sympathetic ganglia, by H.E. stain (slide No. N12)

图6-19   颈交感神经节，HE染色（切片No. N12）

① capsule   ①被膜
② neuron   ②神经元
③ satellite cell   ③卫星细胞
④ lipofuscin pigment   ④脂褐素

| Questions | 问题 |

1.Compare the difference between fibrous and protoplasmic astrocytes.

2.How to identify bundles of nerve fibers from connective tissue?

1.比较纤维型与原浆型星形胶质细胞的差别。

2.如何区分神经纤维束与结缔组织？

Chapter 7　CIRCULATORY SYSTEM

第七章　循环系统

Teaching and Learning Objectives

- To distinguish difference in structural characteristics between arteries and accompanying veins.
- To distinguish difference in structural characteristics between elastic and muscular arteries.
- To identify morphological characteristics of capillaries.
- To identify morphological characteristics of venous valves.
- To identify morphological characteristics of the three layers of heart wall.
- To identify location and morphological characteristics of Purkinje fibers of heart, and to distinguish it from ordinary cardiac muscle cells.

教学目标

- 区分动脉和其伴行静脉的结构特点差异。
- 区分弹性动脉和肌性动脉的结构特点差异。
- 辨认毛细血管的形态特点。
- 辨认静脉瓣的形态特点。
- 辨认心脏壁的3个分层的形态特点。
- 辨认心脏浦肯野纤维的位置和形态特点，区分它与普通心肌细胞的形态差异。

1.Capillaries

(1) Mesentery in whole mount

Arterioles, venules and network of capillaries can be seen in this mount. The nuclei of flattened endothelial cells bulging inward the lumen of capillaries, can be distinguished from those of pericytes bulging outward. Notice the nuclei of smooth muscle lined circumferentially in the arteriole walls (Fig. 7-1).

1.毛细血管

（1）肠系膜铺片

肠系膜铺片中有微动脉、微静脉和毛细血管网。扁平的内皮细胞核凸向管腔，借此可与凸向管外的周细胞核区分。注意微动脉管壁中环形分布的平滑肌细胞核（图7-1）。

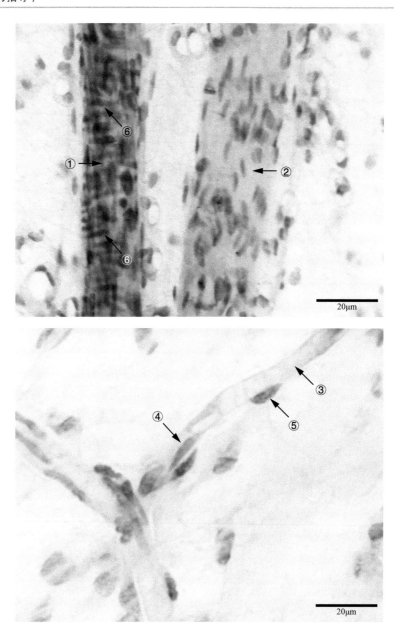

Fig. 7-1　Mesentery in whole mount, by H.E. stain (slide No. Ci1)

图7-1　肠系膜铺片，HE染色（切片No. Ci1）

①arteriole	①微动脉
②venule	②微静脉
③capillary	③毛细血管
④endothelial cell	④内皮细胞
⑤pericyte	⑤周细胞
⑥smooth muscle	⑥平滑肌细胞

(2) Finger skin

Try to find capillary in the dermis just beneath the epithelium, with small lumen to permit passage of one erythrocyte, with flattened endothelial cell nucleus bulging inward lumen (Fig. 7-2).

（2）指皮

在紧挨上皮的真皮中寻找毛细血管，其腔小，仅能容一个红细胞通过，内皮细胞核扁平，突向管腔（图7-2）。

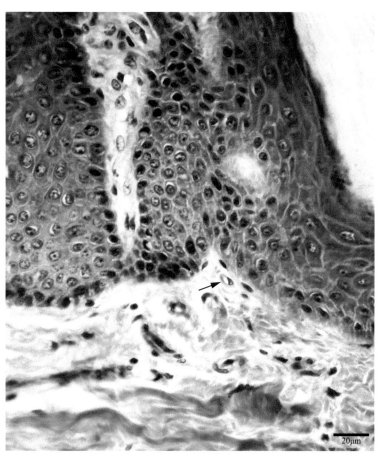

20μm

Fig. 7-2　Finger skin, by H.E stain (slide No. Sk1)
图7-2　指皮，HE染色（切片No. Sk1）

Arrow: capillary　　　　　　　　　　箭头：毛细血管

(3) Liver

Hepatic plate radiates with central vein as core, with sinusoid located among hepatic plates, and lined with non-continuous endothelial cells. Kupffer cells also locates in the sinusoid (Fig. 7-3).

（3）肝

肝板以中央静脉为中心向外放射状发散，血窦位于肝板之间，由不连续的内皮细胞围成，血窦中还有库普弗细胞（图7-3）。

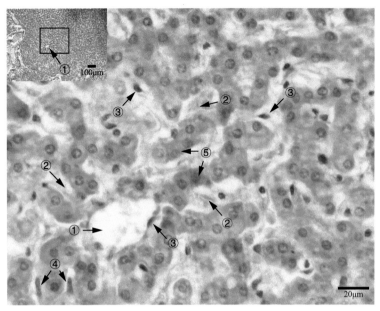

Fig. 7-3　Liver, by H.E. stain (slide No. DG5)
图7-3　肝，HE染色（切片No. DG5）

①central vein　　　　①中央静脉
②sinusoid　　　　　②血窦
③endothelial cell　　③内皮细胞
④Kupffer cell　　　④库普弗细胞
⑤hepatocyte　　　　⑤肝细胞

2.Arterioles and venules

Try to find arterioles and accompanying venules in the interlobular connective tissue. Different from capillary, arteriole has smaller lumen, with one or two layers of smooth muscle cells lined circumferentially in the media of its wall. Venule has a little bit larger and irregular lumen, lack of smooth muscle layer (Fig. 7-4).

2.微动脉和微静脉

在小叶间结缔组织中寻找微动脉及与其伴行的微静脉。微动脉腔小，但管壁中膜中有1～2层呈环形分布的平滑肌细胞。微静脉腔大，管腔不规则，管壁缺乏平滑肌层（图7-4）。

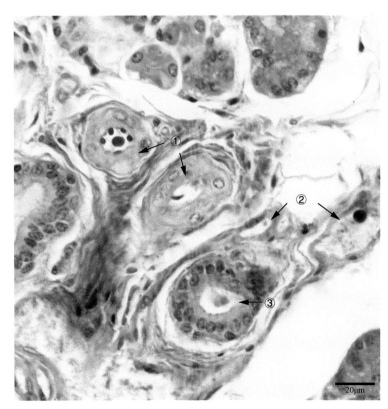

Fig. 7-4　Arterioles and venules, submandibular gland, by H.E. stain (slide No. DG2)
图7-4　微动脉和微静脉，下颌下腺，HE染色（切片No. DG2）

①arteriole　　　　①微动脉
②venule　　　　　②微静脉
③duct　　　　　　③导管

3.Medium-sized artery (muscular artery) and vein

Medium-sized artery has a thinner intima resting upon continuous internal elastic membrane appearing as undulant lining in cross-section. Its media is composed of smooth muscle fibers distributed evenly and circum-

3. 中动脉（肌性动脉）和中静脉

中动脉内膜薄，其外是薄的、横切面上呈波浪状的内弹性膜，中膜是均匀分布的环形平滑肌，外膜与周围结缔组织混杂在一起。

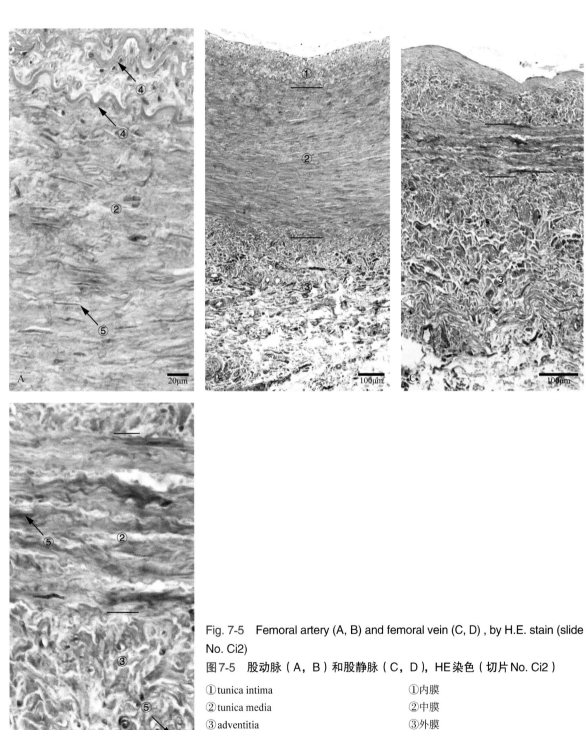

Fig. 7-5　Femoral artery (A, B) and femoral vein (C, D) , by H.E. stain (slide No. Ci2)

图7-5　股动脉（A，B）和股静脉（C，D），HE染色（切片No. Ci2）

①tunica intima	①内膜
②tunica media	②中膜
③adventitia	③外膜
④internal elastic membrane	④内弹性膜
⑤smooth muscle cell	⑤平滑肌细胞

ferentially, and its adventitia blends with the surrounding connective tissue.

Medium-sized vein lacks continuous internal elastic membrane, with very thin media of smooth muscle lined relatively irregularly and interwoven with a substantial amount of connective tissue fibers in adventitia (Fig. 7-5, Fig. 7-6).

中静脉缺乏连续的内弹性膜，中膜很薄，平滑肌分布相对不规则，与外膜大量的结缔组织纤维混杂在一起（图7-5，图7-6）。

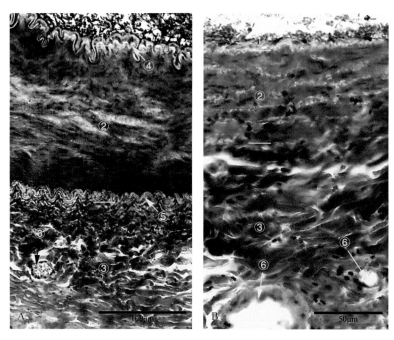

Fig. 7-6　Femoral artery (A) and femoral vein (B)，by azocarmine / R.F. stain (slide No. Ci3)

图7-6　股动脉（A）和股静脉（B），偶氮卡红/醛复红染色（切片No. Ci3）

①tunica intima	①内膜
②tunica media	②中膜
③adventitia	③外膜
④internal elastic membrane	④内弹性膜
⑤external elastic membrane	⑤外弹性膜
⑥vasa vasorum	⑥滋养血管

4.Large artery

Elastic fiber is less in the inner part of tunica intima, and more in its deeper part, having some of endothelial cells lost. Tunica media forms the main part of the wall of large artery, consisted of a large number of elastic membrane mixed with collagenous fibers and smooth muscle cells. Elastic membrane can be seen as deep-stained undulant line in the slide. Boundary between tunica media and tunica intima is not so clear. Tunica adventitia outside media is composed of collagenous fibers and a little of elastic fibers, with vasa vasorum among it (Fig. 7-7).

4.大动脉

弹性纤维在大动脉内膜浅层相对较少而在深层较多，部分内皮细胞可能已经脱落。中膜形成了大动脉壁的主要部分，由大量弹性膜组成，其间混杂着胶原纤维和平滑肌细胞。弹性膜染色较深，呈波浪线状，中膜和内膜的分界不清楚。外膜由胶原纤维和少量弹性纤维组成，其间可见滋养血管（图7-7）。

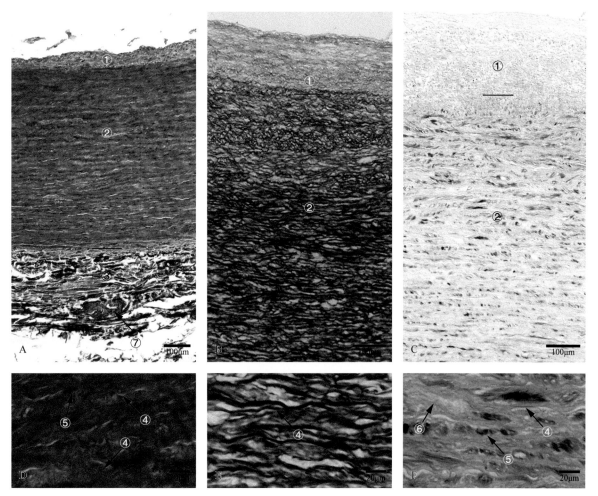

Fig. 7-7　Aorta, by H.E. stain (A, D) (slide No. Ci4) , by R.F. stain (B, E) (slide No. Ci5) , by azocarmine stain (C, F) (slide No. Ci6)
图7-7　主动脉，HE染色（A，D）（切片No.Ci4），醛复红染色（B，E）（切片No.Ci5），偶氮卡红染色（C，F）（切片No.Ci6）

①tunica intima
②tunica media
③adventitia
④elastic membrane
⑤smooth muscle
⑥collagenous fiber
⑦vasa vasorum

①内膜
②中膜
③外膜
④弹性膜
⑤平滑肌细胞
⑥胶原纤维
⑦滋养血管

5.Large vein

Lumen of great vein is large in caliber and irregular in shape with thinner, collapsible wall. Note, in particular, its well-developed adventitia with a few bundles of smooth muscles arranged longitudinally (Fig. 7-8). In addition, valve is an important structural feature of large and medium-sized veins (demonstration slide, Fig. 7-9), which is formed by thin paired folds of tunica intima projecting into the lumen, with connective tissue as core, rich in elastic fibers, and covered with endothelium.

5.大静脉

大静脉腔大，薄壁塌陷而管腔不规则。注意：大静脉发达的外膜中有许多纵形走行的平滑肌束（图7-8）。此外，大静脉和中静脉的一个重要结构特征是有静脉瓣（示教切片，图7-9），由内膜突入管腔折叠而成，其中心为含有弹性纤维的结缔组织，表面覆以内皮。

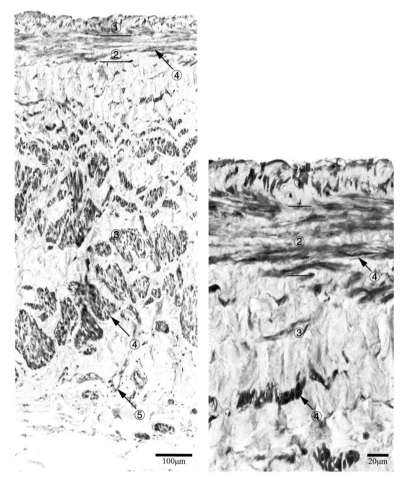

Fig. 7-8　Large vein, by H.E. stain (slide No. Ci7)
图7-8　大静脉，HE染色（切片No. Ci7）

①tunica intima　　　　　　①内膜
②tunica media　　　　　　②中膜
③adventitia　　　　　　　③外膜
④smooth muscle cell　　　④平滑肌细胞
⑤vasa vasorum　　　　　　⑤滋养血管

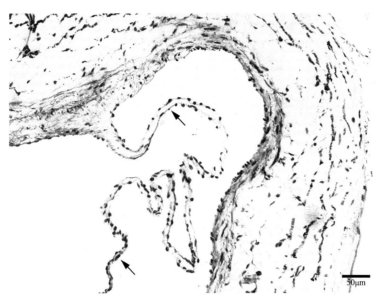

Fig. 7-9   Venous valve in medium-sized vein, by H.E. stain (demonstration slide)

图7-9   静脉瓣，中静脉，HE染色（示教切片）

Arrow: venous valve   箭头：静脉瓣

6.Heart

(1) Heart, from human

First, examine the slide No. Ci8 with naked eyes. The thicker mass in the slide is part of the right ventricular wall and the thinner part linked with the former is pulmonary arterial wall, with valve between them extending laterally and attached to the root of pulmonary artery. Then examine ventricular endocardium under light microscope, inner line of endothelium and outer sub-endothelial connective tissue composed of collagenous and elastic fibers can be seen. The outermost layer of epicardium covered by mesothelium can be seen (but not well preserved in all the slide), rich by adipocytes in connective tissue. Myocardium is composed of large amount of myocardial fibers bundles interwoven longitudinally and vertically. The valve is covered by endothelium, with dense collagenous fibers and elastic fibers as its core (Fig. 7-10).

6.心脏

（1）心脏，人

先用裸眼观察切片No. Ci8，厚的部分是右心室壁，与之相连的薄的部分是肺动脉壁，二者之间侧向突出的是位于肺动脉根部的肺动脉瓣膜。之后，在光镜下观察心内膜，可见内皮和其外由胶原纤维及弹性纤维组成的内皮下结缔组织。心外膜最外层可见间皮覆盖（并非所有切片均可见），其内可见富含脂肪的结缔组织。心肌膜由大量纵横交错、成束排列的心肌纤维组成。瓣膜由内皮覆盖，其核心部分是致密的胶原纤维，也有弹性纤维（图7-10）。

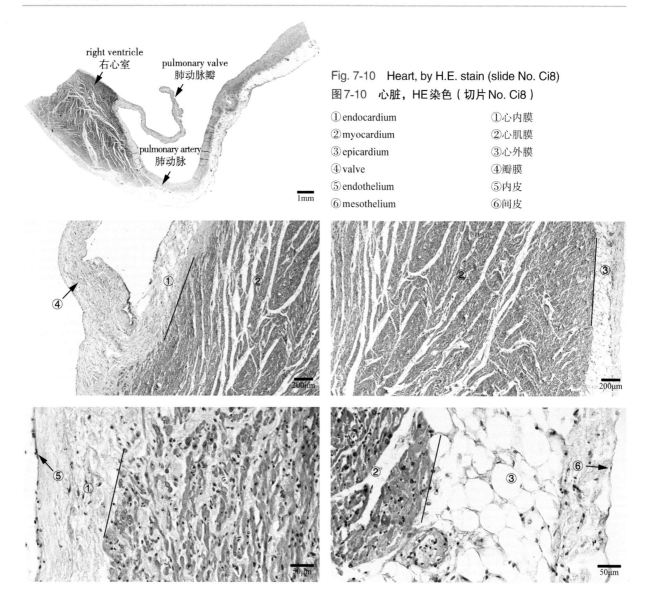

right ventricle
右心室

pulmonary valve
肺动脉瓣

pulmonary artery
肺动脉

1mm

Fig. 7-10　Heart, by H.E. stain (slide No. Ci8)
图7-10　心脏，HE染色（切片 No. Ci8）

① endocardium　　　　　①心内膜
② myocardium　　　　　②心肌膜
③ epicardium　　　　　③心外膜
④ valve　　　　　　　　④瓣膜
⑤ endothelium　　　　　⑤内皮
⑥ mesothelium　　　　　⑥间皮

(2) Heart, from sheep

As observing the subendocardial layer under microscope with low power objective, try to find Purkinje fibers. Examining further its morphological features with high power objective, Purkinje fibers can be seen stained lighter, larger in diameter and fewer myofibrils than those in ordinary myocardial cells (Fig. 7-11).

（2）心脏，绵羊

低倍镜下观察心内膜下层，找到浦肯野纤维，高倍镜下仔细观察其形态，可见与普通心肌细胞相比，它们染色较浅，直径较大，胞质中肌原纤维含量较少（图7-11）。

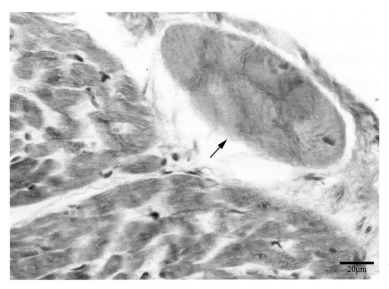

Fig. 7-11   Heart, from sheep, by H.E. stain (slide No. Ci9)
图7-11　心脏，绵羊，HE染色（切片No. Ci9）

Arrow: Purkinje fibers   箭头：浦肯野纤维

7.Lymphatic vessels

Lymphatic vessel is a thinner-wall vessel lined with endothelium, different from vein, without red blood cells in its lumen, but may contain granular lymph and varying numbers of lymphocytes. Valve may also be seen in lymphatic vessel, particularly in longitudinal section (Fig. 7-12).

7.淋巴管

淋巴管是由内皮围成的薄壁管，与静脉不同的是，淋巴管腔中不含红细胞，但其中可有颗粒样的淋巴液和不同数量的淋巴细胞，尤其在纵切面上，常可见到瓣膜（图7-12）。

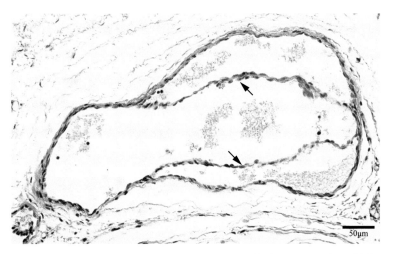

Fig. 7-12   Lymphatic vessel, by azocarmine stain (demonstration slide)
图7-12　淋巴管，偶氮卡红染色（示教切片）

Arrow: valve   箭头：瓣膜

Questions

How to distinguish blood vessel from duct in the light microscope?

问题

如何在光镜下区分血管和导管？

Chapter 8　IMMUNE SYSTEM

第 八 章　免 疫 系 统

Teaching and Learning Objectives

- To recognize cortex and medulla of thymus, as well as Hassall's corpuscles.
- To distinguish lymph nodules (or follicles) from diffused lymph tissue, and to identify germinal center and mantle zone.
- To recognize capsule, hilus, cortex and medulla of lymph nodes, and to identify afferent/efferent lymphatics, high-endothelial venules, macrophages, plasma cells and reticular cells.
- To recognize basic architecture of spleen, including capsule, white and red pulp, and to identify central arteriole and periarteriolar lymphatic sheath.
- To identify tonsil crypts and lymphocytic infiltrated area of epithelium.

教学目标

- 识别胸腺皮质与髓质，辨认胸腺小体。
- 区分淋巴小结（滤泡）与弥散淋巴组织，辨认生发中心与小结帽。
- 识别淋巴结被膜、门部、皮质与髓质结构特征，辨认输入/输出淋巴管，高内皮微静脉，巨噬细胞，浆细胞与网状细胞。
- 识别脾的基本结构：被膜、白髓与红髓，辨认中央动脉及动脉周围淋巴鞘。
- 辨认扁桃体隐窝以及淋巴细胞上皮浸润部。

1.Thymus

Under microscope with low power objective lens, thymus can be seen wrapped by connective tissue capsule which extends inward to subdivide it into incompletely separated lobules. Its cortex is closely adjacent to connective tissue and densely stained, and its medulla locates in the center and stained pale, continuous from lobule to lobule. Cortex consists of lots of T-lymphoblast (or thymocytes) and lightly-stained thymic epithelial cells. The relative preponderance of thymic epithelial cells in medulla, which branch with large nuclei, accounts for its pale appearance, and are difficult to delineate under light microscope, often with one or two prominent nucleoli and distinguishable from thymocytes. Hassall's (or thymus) corpuscle, a unique feature of thymus, can be seen in medulla, with varied size, concentrically lamellate structure, and lightly-stained

1.胸腺

低倍镜下可见胸腺外被结缔组织被膜，向实质内伸入形成小叶间隔，将胸腺分成不完全分隔的小叶。皮质紧挨结缔组织，染色较深；髓质居中，染色较浅，小叶间髓质可相连。皮质由T淋巴母细胞（胸腺细胞）和浅染的胸腺上皮细胞构成。髓质中胸腺上皮细胞相对较多，呈分支状，在光镜下难以辨认细胞轮廓，但细胞核浅色染，常有1～2个明显的核仁，可与胸腺细胞相区分。髓质中还可见胸腺小体，为胸腺的特征性结构，它们体积大小不一，呈同心圆板层状结构，最外层细胞可见浅染细胞核，向内，细胞逐渐角化，胞核消失，胞质呈嗜酸均质状（图8-1）。

nucleus in its outermost layer, but its cells are keratinized gradually as extending inward, with homogeneous acidophilic cytoplasm and disappeared nucleus (Fig. 8-1).

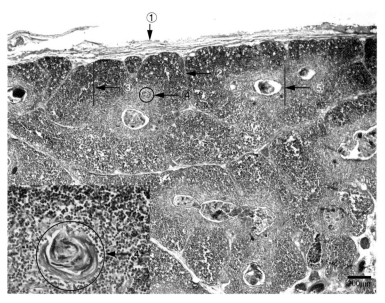

Fig. 8-1　Thymus, from children, by H.E. stain (slide No. Im1)
图8-1　胸腺，儿童，HE染色（切片No. Im1）

①capsule	①被膜
②connective tissue septa	②结缔组织间隔
③cortex	③皮质
④Hassall's corpuscle	④胸腺小体
⑤medulla	⑤髓质

2.Lymph Node

Under microscope with low-power objective lens, outer layer of lymph node is wrapped by a thin connective tissue capsule, which extends inward to form trabecula. In some slides, hilum can be seen at the concave surface of lymph node. Parenchyma of lymph node is composed of densely stained cortex and in-depth lightly stained medulla (Fig. 8-2). More reticular fibers in capsule and trabecula than in parenchyma, serve as supporting framework of lymph node (presenting black thread-shape in silver stain, Fig. 8-3). The plane of afferent lymphatics can be seen in the capsule, with thinner wall and valves, usually no red blood cells in the lumen, therefore, distinguishable from vein. While, efferent lymphatic locates at hilum of lymph node, with similar features as afferent one.

2. 淋巴结

低倍镜下观察，淋巴结外层包被有薄层结缔组织构成的被膜，向实质内延伸形成结缔组织小梁。有些切片淋巴结一侧可见一凹陷，为淋巴结门部。淋巴结实质由浅表的皮质和深部的髓质构成（图8-2）。被膜及小梁中含有较多的网状纤维，实质中也有分布，这些构成了淋巴结的网状支架（银染呈黑色线状，图8-3）。输入淋巴管切面可见于围绕皮质周边的被膜中，管壁薄，腔内可见瓣膜，正常情况下没有红细胞，从而可以与静脉相区别。输出淋巴管特征相同，只是位于淋巴结门部。

Lymphoid nodules (or follicles) distribute discretely in the superficial cortex, mainly composed of B-lymphocytes. The primary lymphoid nodules consists of lymphocytes, as densely-arranged sphere in shape, and light-stain germinal center can be seen in the secondary lymphoid nodules with a small densely-stained mantle zone formed by non-differentiated lymphocytes clustered in one of its sides.

In-depth cortex is composed of diffused lymph tissue, aggregated by large amount of T-lymphocytes, called paracortex, where specialized postcapillary venules (or high endothelial venules, HEV) can be found, with an unusual tall or cuboidal endothelial cells. Small, round, densely-stained nucleus of lymphocyte passing through venule wall, which can often be seen among endothelial cells (Fig. 8-2, Fig. 8-4).

淋巴结皮质浅层分布有淋巴小结（淋巴滤泡），主要由B淋巴细胞构成。HE染色切片上，淋巴细胞密集排列成球形，称为初级淋巴小结，次级淋巴小结中央可见浅染的生发中心，未进入分化的淋巴细胞被推挤在生发中心一侧，形成小结帽。

淋巴小结深部是弥散的淋巴组织，称副皮质区，含大量密集的T淋巴细胞。此区有特殊的毛细血管后微静脉（高内皮细胞微静脉），内皮细胞高或立方形。内皮细胞间常见小而圆且深染的细胞核，为穿越微静脉壁的淋巴细胞（图8-2，图8-4）。

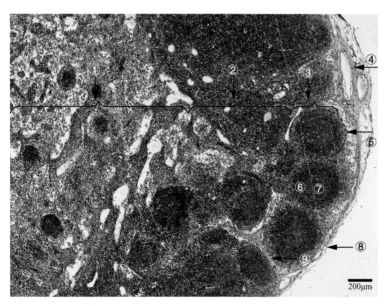

Fig. 8-2　Lymph Node, from rabbit, by H.E. stain (slide No. Im2)

图8-2　淋巴结，兔，HE染色（切片No. Im2）

①medulla	①髓质
②paracortex (in-depth cortex)	②副皮质区（深层皮质）
③superficial cortex	③浅层皮质
④afferent lymphatic	④输入淋巴管
⑤lymphoid nodule	⑤淋巴小结
⑥mantle (corona) zone	⑥小结帽
⑦germinal center	⑦生发中心
⑧capsule	⑧被膜
⑨trabecula	⑨小梁

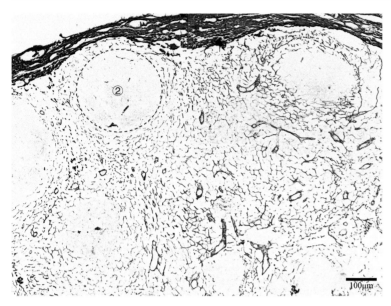

Fig. 8-3 Reticular fibers in lymph node, by silver stain (demonstration slide)

图8-3 淋巴结网状纤维，银染（示教切片）

① capsule   ①被膜
② lymphoid nodule   ②淋巴小结

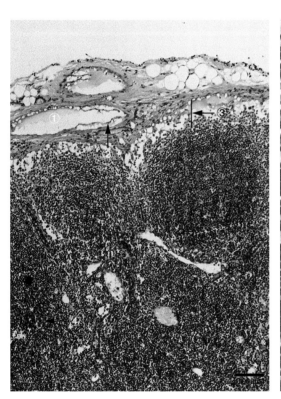
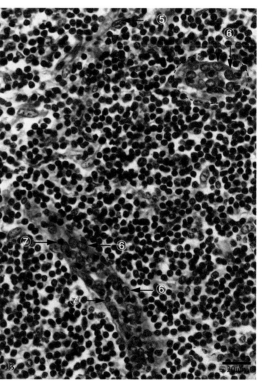

Fig. 8-4 Lymph Node, from rabbit, by H.E. stain (slide No. Im2)

图8-4 淋巴结，兔，HE染色（切片No. Im2）

A.Under low power objective; B.Under high power objective   A.低倍镜；B.高倍镜

① afferent lymphatic   ①输入淋巴管

② valve   ②瓣膜

③ subcapsular sinus   ③被膜下窦

④ HEV   ④高内皮细胞微静脉

⑤ capillary endothelial cell   ⑤普通毛细血管内皮细胞

⑥ endothelial cells of HEV   ⑥HEV内皮细胞

⑦ lymphocytes passing through HEV wall   ⑦穿HEV管壁的淋巴细胞

Irregular arranged lymphoid tissue, continuing from cortex and extending into medulla of lymph nodes, is called medullary cords, between which are medullary sinuses. Reticular cells and reticular fibers constitute the supporting framework of medullary sinuses. Reticular cells can be seen in sinuses, with elliptical and light stained nuclei, sometimes thinner processes. Also, large amount of macrophages can be seen in medullary sinuses, large in size, with round or irregular nuclei, abundant in stronger acidophilic cytoplasm, sometimes containing phagocytosed granules (Fig. 8-5).

与皮质相延续的不规则聚集的淋巴组织深入淋巴结髓质，称为髓索。髓索间为髓窦，髓窦中有网状细胞及网状纤维构成的支架。网状细胞核椭圆，染色浅，有时可见胞质突起。髓窦中还有大量巨噬细胞，体积大，核圆或不规则，胞质丰富，嗜酸性强，有时可见胞质中的吞噬颗粒（图8-5）。

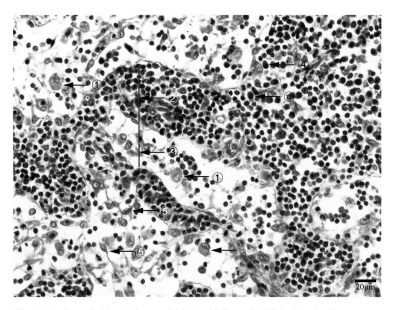

Fig. 8-5 Lymph Node, from rabbit, by H.E. stain (slide No. Im2)
图8-5 淋巴结，兔，HE染色（切片 No. Im2）

①macrophage	①巨噬细胞
②medullary cord	②髓索
③medullary sinus	③髓窦
④plasma cells	④浆细胞
⑤reticular cells	⑤网状细胞

3.Spleen

As observing under microscope with low-power objective, a thick capsule composed of dense connective tissue can be seen in spleen surface, which extends inward the parenchyma to form trabecula, with reticular tissue as its framework (Fig. 8-9). The area densely-stained with concentrated nuclei in parenchyma is called white pulp, and that pink-stained is red pulp (Fig. 8-6). The lymphoid tissue that surrounds central arterioles is called periarteriolar lymphatic sheaths. Occasionally splenic corpuscle (or lymphoid nodule) with germinal center in it can be seen (Fig. 8-7). Red pulp is composed of splenic sinuses and splenic (Billroth's) cords, in which cells, including red blood cells, plasma cells, macrophages, and so on, pack inseparably and difficult to be identified. Macrophage that phagocytosed the aged and frail erythrocytes, containing hemosiderin, can be stained by Prussian blue as greenish-blue (Fig. 8-10). Splenic sinus is surrounded by a layer of elongated epithelial cells, with larger intercellular space, round or triangular nuclei, and outer reticular fibers in cross-section (Fig. 8-8).

3.脾

低倍镜观察脾表面致密结缔组织构成的厚被膜，深入实质形成小梁。小梁间为脾实质，网状组织构成其支架结构（图 8-9）。实质中细胞核密集深染的区域为白髓，粉染区域为红髓（图 8-6）。白髓为围绕中央动脉的淋巴组织，称动脉周围淋巴鞘，偶尔可见带有生发中心的脾小体（淋巴小结）（图 8-7）。红髓由脾血窦和脾索构成。脾索内，含有血细胞、浆细胞、巨噬细胞等，细胞排列紧密不易分辨。由于巨噬细胞吞噬了衰老红细胞，因而胞内含有含铁血黄素颗粒，可被普鲁士蓝染为蓝绿色（图 8-10）。脾血窦由一层长内皮细胞围绕，细胞间隙大，横切面上细胞核呈圆形或三角形，外被网状纤维（图 8-8）。

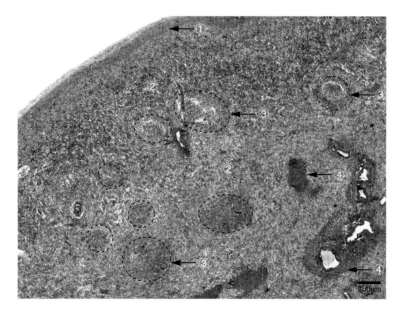

Fig. 8-6　Spleen, from human, by H.E. stain (slide No. Im3)

图 8-6　脾，人，HE 染色（切片 No. Im3）

①capsule	①被膜
②red pulp	②红髓
③white pulp	③白髓
④trabecula	④小梁

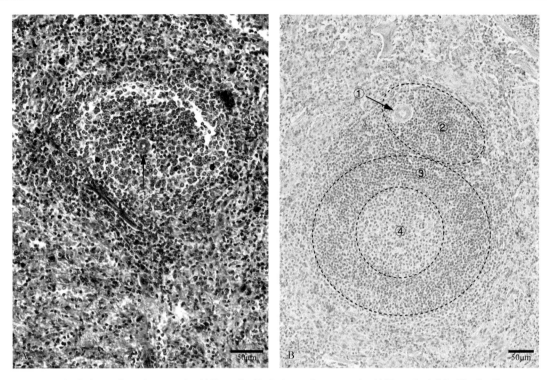

Fig. 8-7　A. Spleen, from human, by H.E. stain; B. Spleen, from cat, by H.E. stain (slide No. Im3)
图 8-7　A. 脾，人，HE 染色；B. 脾，猫，HE 染色（切片 No. Im3）

①central arteriole
②periarteriolar lymphatic sheaths
③mantle zone
④germinal center

①中央动脉
②动脉周围淋巴鞘
③小结帽
④生发中心

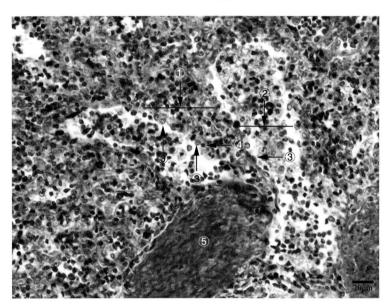

Fig. 8-8　Splenic red pulp, from human, by H.E. stain (slide No. Im3)
图 8-8　脾红髓，人，HE 染色（切片 No. Im3）

①splenic cord
②splenic sinusoid
③endothelial cells
④red blood cell
⑤trabecula

①脾索
②脾血窦
③血窦内皮细胞
④红细胞
⑤小梁

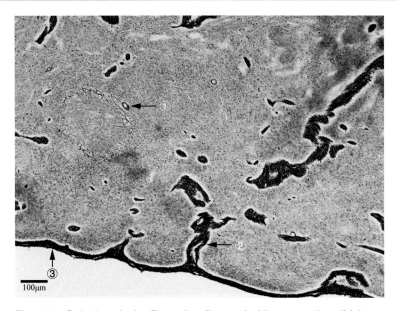

Fig. 8-9　Splenic reticular fibers, by silver stain (demonstration slide)

图8-9　脾网状纤维，银染（示教切片）

①central arteriole　　　　　　　①中央动脉

②trabecula　　　　　　　　　　②小梁

③capsule　　　　　　　　　　　③被膜

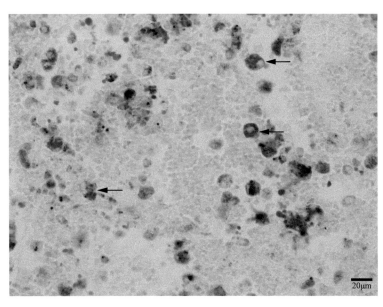

Fig. 8-10　Macrophages, by Prussian blue stain (demonstration slide)

图8-10　脾巨噬细胞，普鲁士蓝染色（示教切片）

Arrow: macrophages　　　　　　箭头：脾巨噬细胞

4.Palatine tonsil

Margin of the palatine tonsil is overlaid by non-keratinized stratificd squamous epithelium, with crypts formed by invaginated epithelia, and often infiltrated by lymphocytes into epithelial cells, which is called intraepithelial infiltration area. Lymphoid nodules and diffused lymphatic tissue can be seen beneath epithelia (Fig. 8-11).

4.腭扁桃体

腭扁桃体一侧被覆未角化的复层扁平上皮，上皮凹陷形成隐窝，此处常有淋巴细胞侵入到上皮细胞间，称上皮浸润部，上皮下为淋巴小结及弥散淋巴组织（图8-11）。

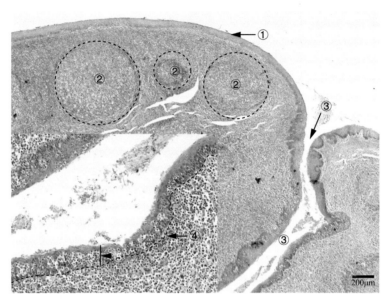

Fig. 8-11　Palatine tonsil, from dog, by H.E. stain (slide No. Im4)
图8-11　腭扁桃体，狗，HE染色（切片No. Im4）

①stratified squamous epithelium	①复层扁平上皮
②lymphoid nodules	②淋巴小结
③crypt	③隐窝
④basement membrane	④基膜
⑤infiltrated epithelium	⑤上皮浸润部

Questions

Compare the common characteristics of lymph node and spleen, as well as their difference.

问题

比较淋巴结和脾的共同特征及区别。

Chapter 9　ENDOCRINE GLANDS

第九章　内分泌腺

Teaching and Learning Objectives

- To identify histological organization of the hypophysis (or pituitary gland), including adenohypophysis (pars distalis, pars intermedia and pars tuberalis) and neuro-hypophysis (pars nervosa, infundibulum).
- To distinguish acidophil, basophil and chromophobe in the pars distalis.
- To identify Herring's body and pituicyte in the pars nervosa.
- To identify thyroid gland, thyroid follicles and follicular epithelial cells.
- To identify parathyroid gland, chief cells and oxyphil cells.
- To identify adrenal gland and to distinguish the similarity and difference in zona glomerulosa, zona fasciculata and zona reticularis, and to identify adrenal medulla.

教学目标

- 辨认垂体的组成部分，包括腺垂体（中间部、远侧部和结节部）和神经垂体（神经部、漏斗）。
- 区分远侧部的嗜酸性细胞、嗜碱性细胞和嫌色细胞。
- 辨认神经部的垂体细胞和赫令体。
- 辨认甲状腺，甲状腺滤泡和滤泡上皮细胞。
- 辨认甲状旁腺，主细胞和嗜酸性细胞。
- 辨认肾上腺，区分肾上腺皮质球状带、束状带、网状带之间的异同；辨认肾上腺髓质。

1.Pituitary gland (hypophysis)

(1) Pituitary gland (longitudinal section)

Slide No. En2 is a sagittal section through the pituitary from monkey. First, observe all portions of the pituitary with naked eyes, i.e., hypothalamus, neurohypophysis and adenohypophysis. Then, under microscope with low power objective, observe the detailed organizations of neurohypophysis and adenohypophysis. The infundibulum of neurohypophysis extends continually from the hypothalamus, with an expanded end as pars nervosa. The adenohypophysis has three parts: the pars distalis is the largest one of it, extending upward the pars tuberalis passing around the stalk of infundibulum in the neurohypophysis, with its adjacent pars intermedia separated from the pars distalis by remnants of Rathke's pouch (not so apparent in some

1.垂体

（1）垂体（纵切）

切片No. En2为猴垂体纵切面，先用肉眼观察垂体各个部分：下丘脑、神经垂体和腺垂体，然后再用低倍镜观察神经垂体和腺垂体的具体结构。神经垂体中的漏斗与下丘脑相延续，其末端膨大为神经部。腺垂体的远侧部是腺垂体最大的一部分，向上延伸的结节部环绕神经垂体的漏斗柄部，中间部则紧贴神经部，其与远侧部间有垂体囊残迹分隔（部分切片不明显）（图9-1）。

slides) (Fig. 9-1).

Observing the pars nervosa in the slide under microscope with high power objective, which consists of large amount of unmyelinated nerve fibers with their cell bodies located in the hypothalamus, i.e., supraoptic nuclei or paraventricular nuclei. Hormones secreted from these neuroendocrine cells deposit locally in the axon as they are transported along it, which form Herring's body, an acidophilic mass can be seen under light microscope. There are a large number of glial cells known as pituicytes. Antidiuretic hormone (ADH) and oxytocin will release into capillaries from the end of the axon, after neuron bodies are stimulated appropriately. A large number of capillaries can be seen in the neurohypophysis. Note to distinguish Herring's bodies from red blood cells in capillaries in the slide.

高倍镜观察此切片的神经部，神经部由大量无髓神经纤维组成，其胞体位于下丘脑的视上核或室旁核中。这些神经内分泌细胞分泌的激素在沿轴突运输的过程中，在轴突局部聚积，形成光镜下可见的均质嗜酸性团块——赫令体。神经纤维之间有大量神经胶质细胞，被称为垂体细胞，抗利尿激素、催产素在神经元胞体受到相应的刺激后，从轴突终末释放，进入毛细血管。在神经垂体中可见大量毛细血管。注意区分赫令体和血管中的红细胞。

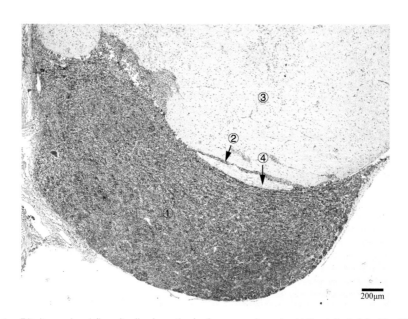

Fig. 9-1　Pituitary gland (longitudinal section), from monkey, by H.E. stain (slide No. En2)

图9-1　垂体（纵切片），猴，HE染色（切片 No. En2）

①pars distalis
②pars intermedia
③pars nervosa
④Rathke's pouch cavity

①远侧部
②中间部
③神经部
④垂体囊腔

(2) Pituitary gland (cross section)

Observe different parts of the pituitary gland in Slide No. En1 under microscope with low power objective, i.e., pars distalis, pars intermedia and pars nervosa (Fig. 9-2A). Then pay more attention to the pars distalis with

（2）垂体（横切）

低倍镜下观察切片 No. En1 横切垂体的远侧部、中间部和神经部（图9-2A），远侧部大量的内分泌细胞排列成团索状，细胞之间有丰富的毛细血管分布，细胞分泌的激素会迅速通

high power objective, where a large number of endocrine cells line up as lumps and cords surrounded by fenestrated capillaries. Hormones secreted by endocrine cells are rapidly transported to the corresponding target organs. Changing to a high-power objective, observe the cells in the pars distalis carefully. Endocrine cells can be divided into chromophils and chromophobes, according to their staining affinity, more chromophobes in quantity, with non-stain or pale-stain in their cytoplasm, sometimes only nucleus can be seen in chromophobes. Chromophils can be divided into acidophilic and basophilic cells according to their staining affinity by H.E. stain. Cytoplasm of acidophil appears bright pink or red by H.E. stain, and that of basophil appears purplish red, with larger body size than that of acidophil. Staining density of their nuclei relates to activation or standstill of their cell function, which is not the basis for distinction of acidophil from basophil (Fig. 9-2C). Acidophil and basophil can be subdivided based on the features of secretory granules in the cells and other characteristics under electron microscope, however, under light microscope which can be distinguished only by immunohistochemical techniques. Follicle structure can be seen in the pars intermedia with varied cells, which is different form thyroid follicle in their constituting cells. Acidophils, basophils and chromophobes all can be involved in the formation of follicle. There is acidophilic colloid material, whose ingredient is unclear, in the follicle cavity (Fig. 9-2B).

There are numerous pituicytes, unmyelinated nerve fibers and acidophilic Herring's bodies distribute in pars nervosa (Fig. 9-2D).

过血液运送到相应的靶器官。换成高倍镜仔细观察远侧部的细胞，内分泌细胞根据其染色情况分为嗜色细胞和嫌色细胞。嫌色细胞数量较多，其胞质不着色或着色很浅，部分嫌色细胞只能观察到细胞核。嗜色细胞在HE染色下根据胞质的染色情况又可分为嗜酸性细胞和嗜碱性细胞，嗜酸性细胞胞质染色鲜红，嗜碱性细胞胞质染色为紫红色、个体较大。细胞核的深染或浅染与细胞功能活跃或静止相关，但这不是嗜酸性、嗜碱性细胞的区分依据（图9-2C）。嗜酸性细胞和嗜碱性细胞的进一步分类是根据电镜下细胞内分泌颗粒特点和其他特征区分的，在光镜下只能通过免疫组化方法区分。

垂体中间部可见滤泡结构存在，与甲状腺滤泡不同，中间部滤泡的构成细胞并不一致，嗜酸性细胞、嗜碱性细胞和嫌色细胞均可参与滤泡构成。滤泡腔中有嗜酸性的胶质存在，其成分不明（图9-2B）。

神经部可见大量垂体细胞，无髓神经纤维和嗜酸性的赫令体分布（图9-2D）。

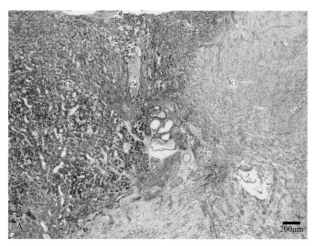

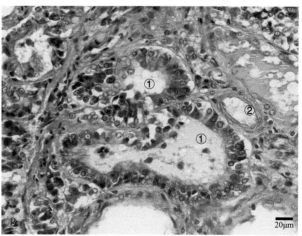

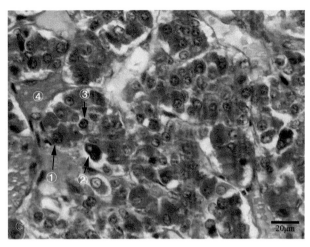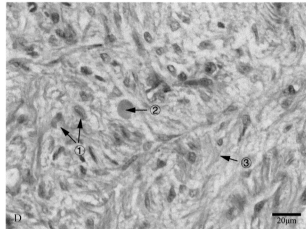

Fig. 9-2　Pituitary gland (cross section), from human, by H.E. stain (slide No. En2)
图9-2　垂体（横切片），人，HE染色（切片No. En2）

A.Low magnification view of the pituitary gland
①pars distalis
②pars intermedia
③pars nervosa
B.Pars intermedia
①follicle
②blood vessel
C.Pars distalis
①acidophil
②basophil
③chromophobe
④capillary
D.Pars nervosa
①pituicyte
②Herring's body
③nerve fiber

A.垂体低倍
①远侧部
②中间部
③神经部
B.中间部
①滤泡
②血管
C.远侧部
①嗜酸性细胞
②嗜碱性细胞
③嫌色细胞
④毛细血管
D.神经部
①垂体细胞
②赫令体
③神经纤维

2.Thyroid gland

Thyroid gland is the only endocrine gland composed of numerous follicles of varied sizes, separated by connective tissue septa with capillaries in it. The follicle is surrounded mostly by cuboidal epithelial cells, flattened or short-columnar in shape depending on their functional status, with acidophilic colloid, homogeneous, pink staining substance, filled in its lumen and with concaved margin in some colloids, which is possibly associated with its reabsorption by epithelial cells. Parafollicular cells are located in the interfollicular space, or involved in follicle composition, but they are difficult to be distinguished with H.E. stain (Fig. 9-3).

2. 甲状腺

甲状腺是唯一一个由大量滤泡组成的内分泌腺，其滤泡数量众多、大小不等，滤泡之间有结缔组织分隔，毛细血管分布于结缔组织中。围成滤泡的滤泡上皮细胞多为立方形，细胞可随功能状态不同变为扁平形或矮柱状。滤泡腔中有嗜酸性的胶质存在，部分胶质边缘呈圆形凹陷，可能与胶质被上皮细胞重吸收有关。滤泡旁细胞分布于滤泡之间，或参与滤泡构成，但在HE染色时很难分辨（图9-3）。

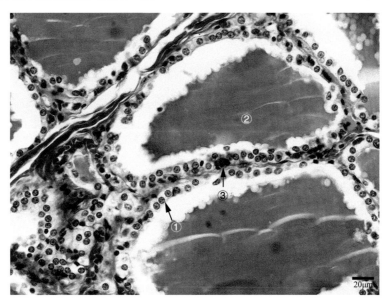

Fig. 9-3   Follicles in thyroid gland, thyroid gland, by H.E. stain (slide No. En4)

图9-3   甲状腺滤泡，甲状腺，HE染色（切片No. En4）

①follicular cells   ①滤泡上皮细胞
②colloid   ②胶质
③capillary   ③毛细血管

3.Parathyroid gland

The parathyroid gland is ovoid in shape and surrounded by capsule. Endocrine cells are arranged in cords or clusters, with rich capillary network among them. The gland contains two types of cells, one is principal (or chief) cell, the other is oxyphil cell. The chief cells are small in size and polygonal in shape, with prominent cellular membrane, centrally-located nucleus and relatively pale and little cytoplasm. Oxyphil cells are scattered in chief cells, or distributed in cluster. The number of oxyphil cells in the parathyroid gland increases with age, which is apparently larger than chief cells, with densely-stained nuclei and strongly eosinophilic cytoplasm (Fig. 9-4).

3. 甲状旁腺

甲状旁腺为椭圆形，外周有被膜包裹。甲状旁腺的内分泌细胞排列成团索状，之间有丰富的毛细血管分布。内分泌细胞主要为主细胞，细胞小呈多角形，细胞膜明显，胞质少、染色浅淡，胞核圆居中。随年龄增加，甲状旁腺内嗜酸性细胞增多，嗜酸性细胞明显比主细胞大，核深染，胞质染成红色。嗜酸性细胞散在分布于主细胞之间或成群分布（图9-4）。

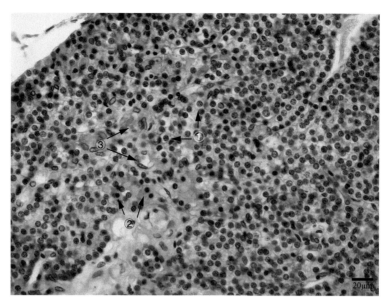

Fig. 9-4　Parathyroid gland, by H.E. stain (slide No. En5)

图9-4　甲状旁腺，HE染色（切片No. En5）

① chief cell	①主细胞
② oxyphil cell	②嗜酸性细胞
③ blood vessel	③血管

4.Adrenal glands

The surface of adrenal gland is covered with thick connective tissue capsule as protective effects. The parenchyma of adrenal gland is divided into two parts, i.e., cortex and medulla (Fig. 9-5), with apparent difference in their embryonic origin, types of hormone secreted and staining affinity. Adrenal cortex can be divided into three zones (or layers).

Zona glomerulosa, lying beneath the capsule, contains cells arranged in spheroid or arch in shape and small in size, with round nuclei and little darker cytoplasm in stain.

Zona fasciculata, the broadest size and lightest-stain in the three zones of cortex, locates in the inner side of zona glomerulosa, and consists of cell cords arranged in parallel, with larger and polyhedral cells, central nuclei, and a large amount of lipid droplets in cytoplasm. As result of dissolution of lipid during tissue preparation, its cytoplasm appears highly vacuolated.

Zona reticularis, the innermost layer adjacent to medulla, is consisted of irregular network of closely packed cells, with smaller in size and more yellowish-brown in stain than those in the zona fasciculata.

4. 肾上腺

肾上腺表面有较厚的结缔组织被膜包裹，起到很好的保护作用。肾上腺的实质分为皮质、髓质两部分（图9-5），两部分在胚胎起源、激素分泌类型、染色等方面均有明显差别。肾上腺皮质分成3层。

球状带，靠近被膜，细胞排列成球形或拱形，细胞较小、染色稍深。

束状带，位于球状带内侧，细胞排列成条索状，束状带细胞较大，胞质内所含的大量脂滴在制片过程中被溶解，使胞质呈现空泡状，束状带在皮质3个带中最宽，染色也最浅。

网状带，最靠近髓质，细胞排列成不规则的网状，网状带细胞较小，胞质呈棕黄色。

The medulla is composed of medullary cells, not sharply delimited from the cortex. Epinephrine-and norepinephrine-producing cells of the medulla can not be distinguished by routine H.E. stain. Medullary cells appear polygonal in shape, larger in size, and weaker basophilic cytoplasm than those in the zona reticularis. As fixed with chromic salt, catecholamines in the secretory granules of cytoplasm in the medullary cells are oxidized as yellowish-brown in color, referred to chromaffin cells (Fig. 9-6A). Single neuron cell or cluster of ganglion cells can also be found in the medulla. Neuron appear obviously larger in size than medullary cells, with round nuclei, prominent nucleoli and basophilic cytoplasm, and are surrounded by satellite cells, occasionally (Fig. 9-6B).

A large number of capillaries can be seen in the cortex and medulla as well as larger medullary central venules in the medulla.

肾上腺髓质由髓质细胞构成，分泌肾上腺素的细胞和分泌去甲肾上腺素的细胞在HE染色时无法区分。髓质细胞呈多角形，个体较皮质网状带细胞大，胞质较多，呈弱嗜碱性。当用铬盐固定时，胞质分泌颗粒中的儿茶酚胺类物质被氧化，使胞质呈现棕黄色，因此髓质细胞也被称为嗜铬细胞（图9-6A）。在髓质中还能观察到神经元细胞单个或成群分布，神经元细胞个体明显比髓质细胞大，核圆且核仁明显，胞质嗜碱，细胞周围偶见卫星细胞包裹（图9-6B）。

皮质与髓质都可观察到大量毛细血管，髓质中还可观察到较大的髓质中央静脉。

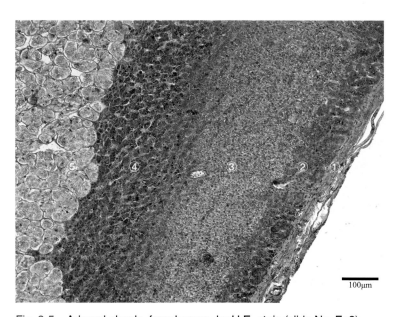

100μm

Fig. 9-5　Adrenal glands, from human, by H.E. stain (slide No. En3)
图9-5　肾上腺，人，HE染色（切片No. En3）

①capsule
②zona glomerulosa
③zona fasciculata
④zona reticularis
⑤medulla

①被膜
②球状带
③束状带
④网状带
⑤髓质

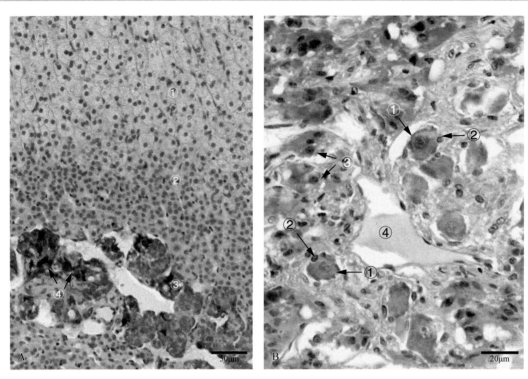

Fig. 9-6 Medulla of adrenal glands (demonstration slide)
图9-6 肾上腺髓质（示教切片）

A.Chromaffin cells, fixed with chromic salts, by H.E. stain

①zona fasciculata

②zona reticularis

③medulla

④chromaffin cells

B.Ganglion cells, from human, by H.E. stain

①ganglion cells

②satellite cell

③medullary cells

④blood vessel

A.嗜铬细胞，铬盐固定，HE染色

①束状带

②网状带

③髓质

④嗜铬细胞

B.神经节细胞，人，HE染色

①神经元

②卫星细胞

③髓质细胞

④血管

Questions

How to distinguish an endocrine organ from the other organs, such as lymphatic organs, exocrine glands?

问题

内分泌器官如何与其他器官区别，如淋巴器官、外分泌腺？

Chapter 10　SKIN and TONGUE

第十章　皮肤和舌

Teaching and Learning Objectives

- To identify stratification of the skin, as well as that of thick and thin epidermis.
- To identify structural features of skin appendages: hair follicles (hair bulb, inner and outer root sheaths), sebaceous gland and sweat gland (to distinguish acini from duct, and to identify myoepithelial cells).
- To identify Meissner corpuscle and Pacinian corpuscle.
- To compare difference in the structure of skin covering varied regions of the body.
- To identify four types of papillae in the surface of tongue: filiform, fungiform, circumvallate and foliate papillae.
- To identify taste buds including gustatory cells, supporting cells and basal cells.

教学目标

- 辨认皮肤层次，以及厚表皮、薄表皮的层次。
- 辨认皮肤附属器的结构特征：毛囊（毛球，内外根鞘）、皮脂腺和汗腺（区分腺泡与导管，辨认肌上皮细胞）。
- 辨认触觉及环层小体。
- 区分不同部位皮肤的结构差别。
- 辨认4种舌乳头，丝状乳头、菌状乳头、轮廓乳头、叶状乳头。
- 辨认味蕾，包括味细胞、支持细胞和基底细胞。

1.Skin in finger tip

Try to observe three-layer structure of skin under microscope with low power objective: the epidermis, the stronger basophilic epithelial tissue region and the dermis composed of irregular dense connective tissue with numerous blood vessels, nerves, sweat glands, and encapsulated nerve endings, et al., and the hypodermis (or subcutaneous tissue) with connective tissue containing more adipose tissue (Fig. 10-1).

Try to observe thick epidermis under microscope with high power objective: the stratum basale composed of a layer of heavy basophilic cuboidal cells attached to basement membrane, with densely arranged nuclei; the stratum spinosum, with cells in this layer appearing large in size, from polygonal to flattened in shape,

1.指皮

低倍镜下观察皮肤的3层结构：嗜碱性较强的上皮组织区域为表皮；不规则致密结缔组织构成真皮，其间分布有大量血管、神经、汗腺、有被囊的神经末梢等；有较多脂肪组织分布的结缔组织为皮下层（图10-1）。

高倍镜下观察厚表皮：厚表皮紧贴基膜，细胞核排列密集，胞质嗜碱性强的一层为基底层；棘层细胞体积增大，从多边形逐渐过渡到扁平，细胞核大而圆，细胞间可见到细胞突起，称细胞间桥；颗粒层细胞3～5层，形状扁平，胞质内含大量强嗜碱性颗粒；透明层在

round and big nuclei, and intercellular spikes referred to "intercellular bridges"; the stratum granulosum, with thrcc-to five-layer flattened cells, flat round nuclei, and numerous basophilic granules; the stratum lucidum, not so apparently in this slide (Fig. 10-3); with thicker stratum corneum, flattened cells, homogeneous cytoplasm and devoid of nuclei (Fig. 10-2).

Dermal connective tissue protrudes into epidermis forming the dermal papillae, with less fibrous components and numerous capillaries, called papillary layer. Sometimes, Meissner corpuscle can be seen in dermal papillae (Fig. 6-14); irregular dense connective tissue beneath dermal papillae layer forms dermal reticular layer with coarse and large collagenous fibers; and Pacinian corpuscles and sweat gland can be seen in the slide. Try to identify acini and duct of sweat gland: small lumen acini are lined with light stained epithelial cells with round nuclei, enclosed by acidophilic basement membrane. Flat or triangular nuclei from myoepithelial cells, sometimes surrounded by acidophilic cytoplasm, locate just inside the basement membrane, while nuclei from fibroblasts locate outside. Ducts of sweat glands are stained dark than acini, with small dark stained nuclei arranging closely into multilayer. Observe their coiled passage through dermis and epidermis and terminally opening on skin surface (Fig. 10-4).

此张切片不明显；但可见厚的角化层，细胞扁平，均质状，细胞核消失（图10-2）特染的透明层见图10-3。

真皮结缔组织向表皮方向突起形成真皮乳头，此处纤维成分较少，称乳头层，含大量毛细血管，乳头内有时可见触觉小体（图6-14）；乳头层深部不规则致密结缔组织为真皮网织层，胶原纤维粗大，网状排列，可见环层小体及汗腺。辨认汗腺腺泡及导管：腺泡染色浅，腺腔小，上皮细胞核圆形，外周嗜酸性基膜明显，紧贴基膜内部可见长椭圆或三角形细胞核，有时周围有嗜酸性胞质，为肌上皮细胞，而成纤维细胞位于基膜外。汗腺导管染色深，细胞多层，排列紧密，细胞核小染色深，弯曲走行，最终开口于皮肤表面（图10-4）。

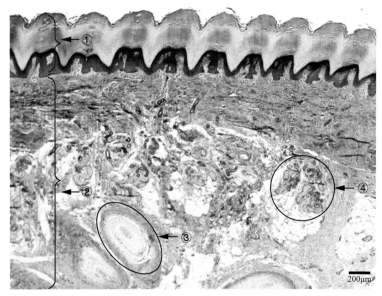

Fig. 10-1　Skin in finger tip, from human, by H.E. stain (slide No. Sk1)

图 10-1　指皮，人，HE染色（切片No. Sk1）

①epidermis　　　　　　①表皮
②dermis　　　　　　　②真皮
③Pacinian corpuscle　　③环层小体
④sweat gland　　　　　④汗腺

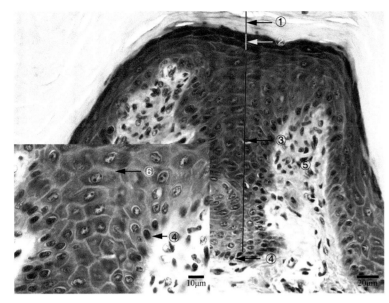

Fig. 10-2   Skin in finger tip, from human, by H.E. stain (slide No. Sk1)

图10-2   指皮，人，HE染色（切片 No. Sk1）

① stratum corneum and stratum lucidum	①角化层与透明层
② stratum granulosum	②颗粒层
③ stratum spinosum	③棘层
④ stratum basale	④基底层
⑤ dermal papillae	⑤真皮乳头
⑥ intercellular bridges	⑥细胞间桥

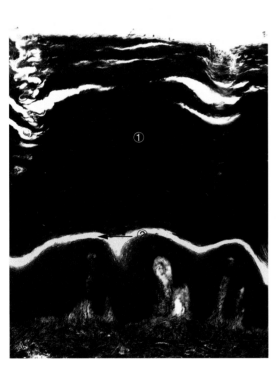

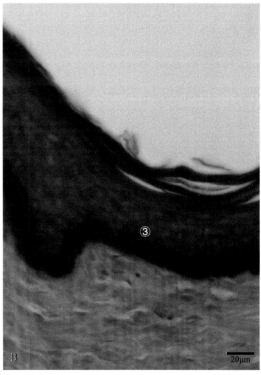

Fig. 10-3   Skin in finger tip, from human, by H.E. stain (demonstration slide)

图10-3   指皮，人，HE染色（示教切片）

A. Thick epidermis in palm from human, by triple stain;

B. Thin epidermis from black people's skin, by H.E. stain

① stratum corneum

② stratum lucidum

③ stratum basale with many melanin granules

A. 手掌厚表皮，人，三色染色；

B. 黑种人薄表皮，HE染色

①角化层

②透明层

③含许多黑素颗粒的基底层

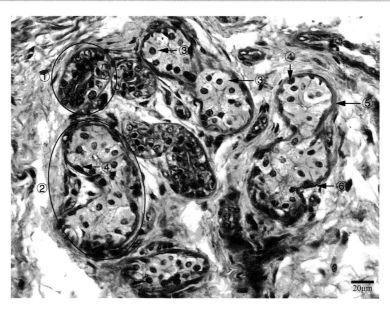

Fig. 10-4   Skin in finger tip, from human, by H.E. stain (slide No. Sk1)

图10-4   指皮，人，HE染色（切片No. Sk1）

①duct of sweat gland
②acini of sweat gland
③secretory cell
④myoepithelial cell
⑤basement membrane
⑥fibroblast

①汗腺导管
②汗腺腺泡
③分泌细胞
④肌上皮细胞
⑤基膜
⑥成纤维细胞

2.Skin

Compare the difference in stratum-specific structure between thin epidermis from human and thick epidermis of finger tip skin (Fig. 10-5). Stratum basale contains more pigment granules, particularly in skin of black people (Fig. 10-3). Note that not all these cells which contain pigment granules are melanocytes.

2.体皮

比较人体皮的薄表皮与指皮厚表皮间各层结构的差别（图10-5）。基底层含色素较多，黑种人皮肤更为明显（图10-3）。注意含有色素的细胞并非全部为黑素细胞。

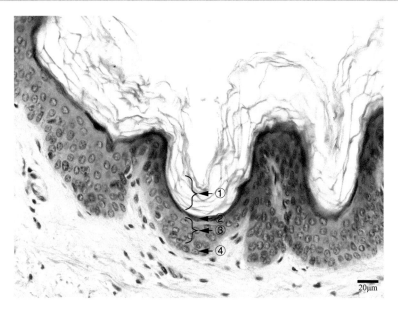

Fig. 10-5   Skin, from human, by H.E. stain (slide No. Sk2)
图10-5   体皮，人，HE染色（切片No. Sk2）

①stratum corneum   ①角化层
②stratum granulosum   ②颗粒层
③stratum spinosum   ③棘层
④stratum basale   ④基底层

3.Scalp

There are many hair follicles in scalp. Try to identify the basic structure of hair root and hair follicle. Observe the structure of hair bulb at the bottom of hair follicle, which is composed of central connective tissue (hair papilla) and peripheral stronger basophilic hair matrix cells. Melanocytes among them give hair color, but which cannot be distinguished by H.E. stain (Fig. 10-6).

Observe structure of hair follicle lining at upper hair bulb, with the outermost layer composed of connective tissue called connective tissue sheath, inner connective tissue sheath is epidermal root sheath composed of epidermal cells, and the innermost hair root composed of keratinized epithelial cells. Epidermal root sheath can be divided into two layers, the inner one called internal root sheath, with strong acidophilic, transparent hair matrix granules, and the outer one called external root sheath, with densely arranged epidermal cells, like spinal layer and basal layer of the epidermis (Fig. 10-7).

Sebaceous gland can be seen attached to the upper hair follicle, where internal root sheath structure gradually disappeared. Acinus of sebaceous gland stains light,

3.头皮

头皮中含有较多毛囊。辨认毛根、毛囊的基本结构并观察毛囊底部的毛球结构，毛球中央为结缔组织构成的毛乳头，周围为毛母质细胞，细胞排列密集，嗜碱性较强，细胞间可有黑素细胞分布，赋予毛发颜色，但在HE染色切片中不易分辨（图10-6）。

在毛球上部观察毛囊层次结构，最外为结缔组织构成的结缔组织根鞘，向内为上皮细胞构成的上皮根鞘，最内是角化细胞构成的毛根。上皮根鞘又分为2层，内层称内根鞘，其上皮细胞内含有强嗜酸的透明毛质颗粒；外层类似表皮的棘层及基底层，为密集排列的上皮细胞（图10-7）。

毛囊上部，内根鞘结构逐渐消失，外周可见皮脂腺。皮脂腺腺泡染色浅淡，外层细胞小，为皮脂腺中的干细胞。向内细胞体积增

with small outer cells as its stem cells, and big sized inner cells with round nuclei and foam-like cytoplasm. In the process gradually approaching to duct, cells collapse, nuclei shrink and deform, and finally are expelled with secretion. Duct of sebaceous gland is shorter with an opening at the upper hair follicle (Fig. 10-8).

A bundle of smooth muscle can be seen beneath sebaceous gland, extending from hair follicle to epithelia, referred to arrector pili muscles (Fig. 5-9, Fig. 10-6).

大，核圆，胞质泡沫状。在逐渐靠近导管的过程中，细胞崩解，细胞核固缩变形，最终随分泌物一起排出。皮脂腺导管短，开口于毛囊上部（图 10-8）。

皮脂腺下方可见一束平滑肌，从毛囊延伸到表皮下，为立毛肌（图 5-9，图 10-6）。

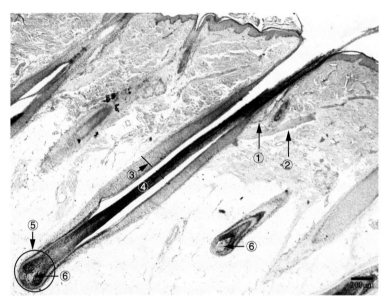

Fig. 10-6　Scalp, from human, by H.E. stain (slide No. Sk3)
图 10-6　头皮，人，HE染色（切片 No. Sk3）

① sebaceous gland	① 皮脂腺
② arrector pili muscle	② 立毛肌
③ hair follicle	③ 毛囊
④ hair root	④ 毛根
⑤ hair bulb	⑤ 毛球
⑥ hair papilla	⑥ 毛乳头

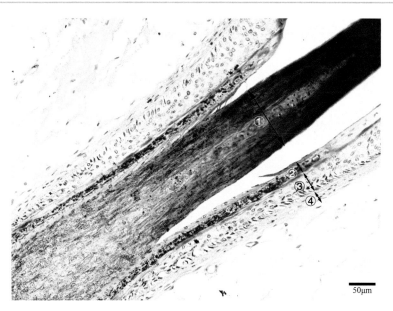

Fig. 10-7　Scalp, from human, by H.E. stain (slide No. Sk3)
图 10-7　头皮，人，HE 染色（切片 No. Sk3）

①hair root　　　　　　　　　　①毛根
②internal (inner) root sheath　　②内根鞘
③external (outer) root sheath　　③外根鞘
④connective tissue sheath　　　④结缔组织鞘

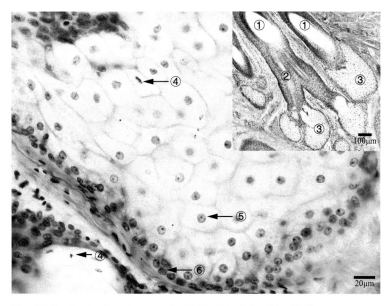

Fig. 10-8　Scalp, from human, by H.E. stain (slide No. Sk3)
图 10-8　头皮，人，HE 染色（切片 No. Sk3）

①hair follicle　　　　　　　　　　　①毛囊
②duct of sebaceous gland　　　　　　②皮脂腺导管
③acini of sebaceous gland　　　　　　③皮脂腺腺泡
④shrunk nuclei of secretary cell (acinic　④皮脂腺细胞固缩的细胞核
　cell) of sebaceous gland
⑤secretary cell of sebaceous gland　　⑤皮脂腺细胞
⑥basal cell of sebaceous gland　　　　⑥皮脂腺基底细胞

4.Tongue

Under microscope with low power objective, the surface of tongue lines with stratified squamous keratinized epithelium, with numerous papillary projects (i.e., filiform, fungiform, foliate and circumvallate papillae) at the dorsal surface of tongue. Core of the tongue consists of intersecting skeletal muscle fibers, intermingled with a few salivary glands.

Try to identify filiform papilla in slide No. DT1: numerous conical shaped processes formed by epithelium and lamina propria, presenting triangular shape in the slide, with heavily keratinized stratified squamous epithelium.

Identify fungiform papilla in slide No. DT2: mushroom-like large processes formed by epithelium and lamina propria, with pale stain oval region among epithelial cells found at its apical surface, where taste buds locate.

Identify circumvallate papilla in slide No. DT3: large mushroom-like prominences formed by non-keratinized stratified squamous epithelium and lamina propria, surrounded by deep moat-like groove, with small serous salivary glands at its bottom, referred to taste gland or gland of von Ebner (with an opening within the surrounded groove), and taste buds at its lateral surface.

See foliate papilla in the demonstration slide: several arch-shape papillary prominences with connective tissue papillae lined in parallel, and taste buds at its lateral surface (Fig. 10-9).

4.舌

低倍镜下可见舌表面被覆一层复层扁平上皮。舌背有乳头状突起，为丝状、菌状、叶状及轮廓乳头。舌体中央为交叉排列的骨骼肌，之间有少量小唾液腺。

切片No. DT1上辨认丝状乳头：上皮和固有层结缔组织向上形成锥形隆起，切面上呈三角形，上皮高度角化。

切片No. DT2上辨认菌状乳头：上皮和固有层结缔组织向上形成蘑菇形隆起，游离面有时可见细胞间浅染椭圆形区域，为味蕾所在。

切片No. DT3上辨认轮廓乳头：上皮和固有层形成巨大的蘑菇状隆起，周围有深的环沟，沟底周围可见小浆液性唾液腺，为味腺，又称von Ebner腺，开口于环沟内。上皮不角化，乳头侧面上皮细胞间可见味蕾。

叶状乳头见示教切片，多个拱形隆起的乳头状突起，结缔组织乳头平行排列，侧面可见味蕾（图10-9）。

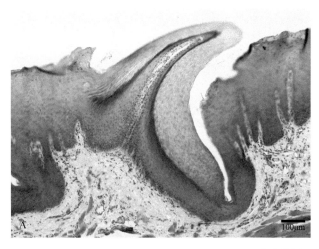
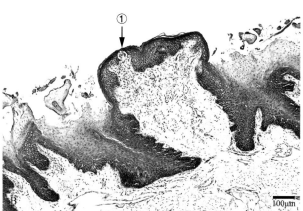
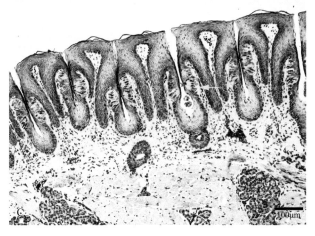
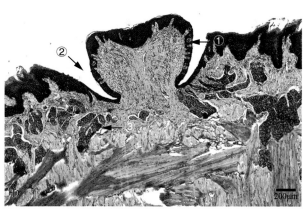

Fig. 10-9   Tongue
图 10-9　舌

A. Filiform papilla of tongue, from cat, by H.E. stain (slide No. DT1)

B. Fungiform papilla of tongue, from monkey, by H.E. stain (slide No. DT2)

C. Foliate papilla of tongue, from rabbit, by I.H. stain (demonstration slide)

D. Circumvallate papilla of tongue, from monkey, by H.E. stain (slide No. DT3)

① taste bud

② surrounded groove (or sulcus, furrow)

③ gland of von Ebner

A. 丝状乳头，猫，HE 染色（切片 No. DT1）

B. 菌状乳头，猴，HE 染色（切片 No. DT2）

C. 叶状乳头，兔，IH 染色（示教切片）

D. 轮廓乳头，猴，HE 染色（切片 No. DT3）

① 味蕾

② 环沟

③ 味腺

Try to identify taste buds under microscope with high power objective: ovoid body extending throughout the full thickness of epithelium, lightly-stained, sometimes with an opening at the surface of epithelium, known as taste pore. That with large, round nucleus and loose chromatin is gustatory cell, that with dense chromatin is supporting cell and that with nucleus close to the basement membrane is basal cell (Fig. 10-10).

高倍镜下辨认味蕾内细胞结构：味蕾跨越上皮全层，浅染，椭圆形结构，有时可见开口于上皮表面，即味孔。其中胞核大，椭圆，染色质疏松的为味细胞，核染色质致密的为支持细胞，胞核位置贴近基膜的为基细胞（图10-10）。

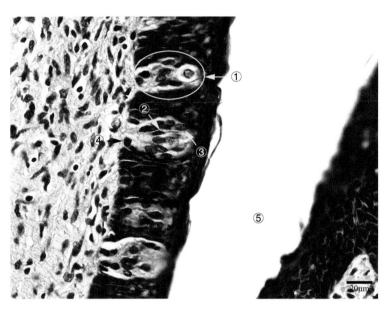

Fig. 10-10　Circumvallate papilla of tongue, from monkey, by H.E. stain (slide No. DT 3)

图10-10　轮廓乳头，猴，HE染色（切片No. DT3）

① taste bud	① 味蕾
② supporting cell	② 支持细胞
③ gustatory cell	③ 味细胞
④ basal cell	④ 基细胞
⑤ surrounded groove	⑤ 环沟

Questions

Which layer shows the most changes as comparing the thick and thin epidermis?

问题

厚表皮与薄表皮，哪层变化最大？

Chapter 11　DIGESTIVE GLANDS

第十一章　消　化　腺

Teaching and Learning Objectives

- To identify the basic structure of digestive gland: secretory acini including serous acini, mucous acini and mixed acini; and duct system including intercalated ducts, striated ducts, intralobular ducts and interlobular ducts.
- To distinguish three pairs of salivary glands: parotid gland, submandibular gland and sublingual gland.
- To identify pancreas, to distinguish its exocrine portion from endocrine portion, to identify the structure of varied parts of exocrine portion, including acini, centroacinar cells, intercalated ducts, etc. And to list the types of endocrine cells in pancreatic islet and their location.
- To identify liver, components of the liver lobule, including central vein, hepatic sinusoids, hepatic cords and portal area.To identify the structure of portal area, including interlobular arterioles, interlobular venules, and interlobular bile ducts, and to identify hepatocytes and Kupffer's cells (hepatic macrophages).
- To identify gallbladder.

教学目标

- 辨认消化腺的基本结构，即腺泡和导管。腺泡包括浆液性、黏液性和混合性腺泡，导管包括闰管、纹状管、小叶内导管和小叶间导管。
- 区分3大唾液腺：腮腺、下颌下腺和舌下腺。
- 辨认胰腺，区分内分泌部和外分泌部。辨认胰腺外分泌部各结构，包括腺泡、泡心细胞、闰管等，列出胰岛内分泌细胞的种类和分布位置。
- 辨认肝脏及肝小叶的组成部分，包括中央静脉、肝血窦、肝索、门管区；辨认门管区的结构，包括小叶间动脉、静脉和小叶间胆管；辨认肝细胞和库普弗细胞（肝巨噬细胞）。
- 辨认胆囊。

1.Parotid gland

Parotid gland is subdivided into many lobules by connective tissue septa, where interlobular ducts, blood vessels and nerves can be seen, and epithelia of interlobular ducts spread from single stratum to stratified gradually. Acini and intralobular ducts at varied levels can be seen in the parotid lobules. Adipocytes increase gradually with age. All parotid acini are serous, with round nuclei near its base and stronger basophilic cytoplasm surrounded, and their acidophilic secretory granules at the apical part of cells are usually dissolved in preparation of the slide. The flattened myoepithelial cells can be seen at

1.腮腺

腮腺被结缔组织分隔成多个小叶，小叶间隔中可见小叶间导管、血管、神经等走行，小叶间导管上皮逐渐从单层向复层过渡。腮腺的小叶内可见腺泡和各级小叶内的导管，随着年龄增加小叶中的脂肪细胞逐渐增加。腮腺的腺泡均为浆液性腺泡，腺细胞核圆近基底部，核周的胞质嗜碱性较强，细胞顶部的嗜酸性分泌颗粒常在制片过程中溶解消失。腺泡基底面有肌上皮细胞，HE染色时很难辨认。与腺泡相连的导管称闰管，由单层立方上皮构成其管壁，

the base of acini, which are difficult to be found in H.E. stain. The duct connecting with acini is called intercalated duct, composed of simple cuboidal epithelium as its wall with small lumen at the center and pale stain cytoplasm. Epithelium of the striated duct is composed of simple columnar epithelial cells, with obviously enlarged lumen and acidophilic cytoplasm, and sometimes vertical striae at its base (Fig. 11-1).

中央的管腔小，闰管上皮细胞胞质染色浅淡。纹状管上皮为单层柱状上皮，管腔明显增大，纹状管细胞胞质嗜酸性，基底部有时可见纵纹（图11-1）。

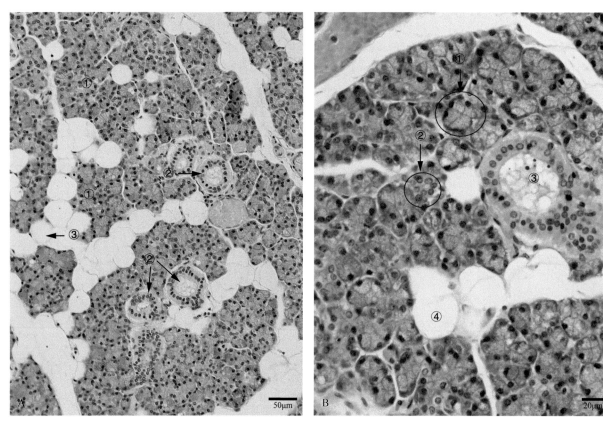

Fig. 11-1　Parotid, by H.E. stain (slide No. DG1)
图 11-1　腮腺，HE 染色（切片 No DG1）

A.Under low power objective
①secretory acini
②ducts
③adipocytes
B.Under high power objective
①serous acini
②intercalated duct
③striated duct
④adipocytes

A.低倍镜
①分泌部
②导管
③脂肪细胞
B.高倍镜
①浆液性腺泡
②闰管
③纹状管
④脂肪细胞

2.Submandibular gland

In submandibular gland, three types of acini can be seen, i.e., serous, mucous and mixed acini, with serous acini accounted for the largest proportion. Round nucleus of serous cell is located near its base, with weaker basophilic cytoplasm

2. 下颌下腺

下颌下腺可见3种腺泡，即浆液性、黏液性和混合性腺泡，其中浆液性腺泡在下颌下腺所占比例最大。浆液性腺细胞核圆，位于细胞的近基底部，周围胞质呈嗜碱性；黏液性腺细

surrounded. Flattened nucleus of mucous cell attaches to its base, with foamy-appearing cytoplasm due to dissolution of mucous secretory granules in it during preparation of the slide. Mixed acini are composed of both mucous cells and serous cells, with darker stain serous cells aggregated at one side of the mixed acini, referred to serous demilune. Sometimes, plasma cells can be seen in surrounding connective tissue. Intralobular ducts of the submandibular gland include both intercalated and striated ducts, with pale stain cytoplasm and smaller lumen in intercalated ducts, and acidophilic cytoplasm in striated ducts (Fig. 11-2).

胞核扁，贴在细胞基底部，胞质内所含的黏原性分泌颗粒制片时被溶解，使胞质呈泡沫状；混合性腺泡由黏液性腺细胞和浆液性腺细胞共同构成，染色较深的浆液性腺细胞聚在一起，位于混合性腺泡的一侧，该结构称为浆半月。有时腺泡之间的结缔组织中可见浆细胞。下颌下腺中小叶内导管既有闰管又有纹状管，闰管胞质染色浅淡，管腔较小，纹状管胞质呈嗜酸性（图11-2 ）。

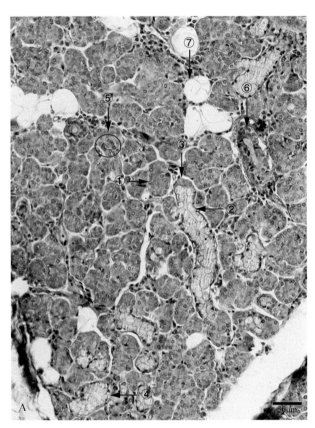
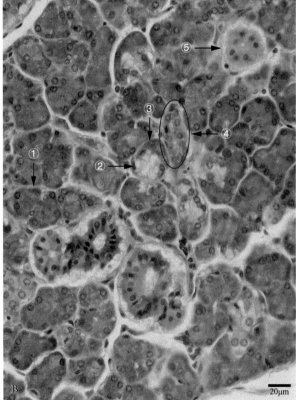

Fig. 11-2　Submandibular gland, by H.E. stain (slide No. DG2)
图11-2　下颌下腺，HE染色（切片No. DG 2 ）

A.Under low power objective
①serous acinus
②mixed acinus
③serous demilune
④mucous acinus
⑤intercalated duct
⑥striated duct
⑦adipocytes
B.Under high power objective
①serous acinus
②mixed acinus
③serous demilune
④intercalated duct
⑤striated duct

A.低倍镜
①浆液性腺泡
②混合性腺泡
③浆半月
④黏液性腺泡
⑤闰管
⑥纹状管
⑦脂肪细胞
B.高倍镜
①浆液性腺泡
②混合性腺泡
③浆半月
④闰管
⑤纹状管

3.Sublingual gland

Sublingual gland is mainly composed of mucous and mixed acini, with less intralobular ducts, and the interlobular ducts are surrounded by prominent connective tissue (Fig. 11-3).

3. 舌下腺

舌下腺内以黏液性和混合性腺泡为主，小叶内的导管较少，小叶间导管周围有明显的结缔组织（图11-3）。

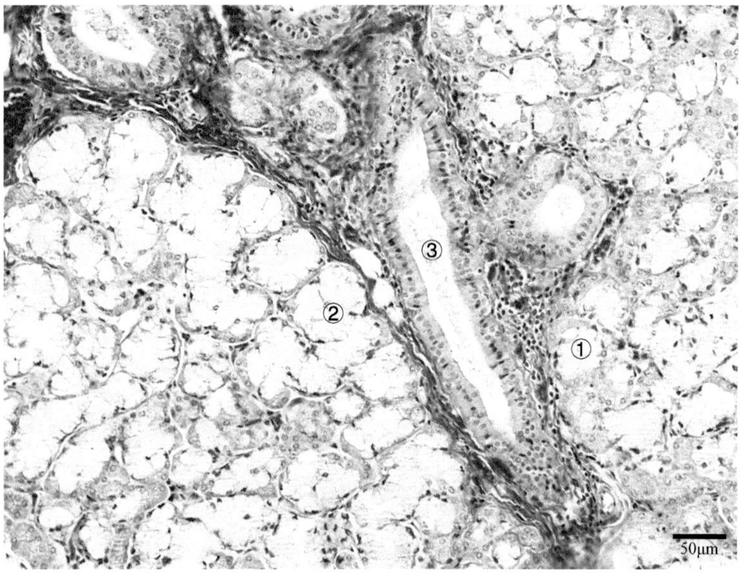

Fig. 11-3 Sublingual gland, by H.E. stain (slide No. DG3)

图11-3 舌下腺，HE染色（切片No. DG3）

①mixed acinus	①混合性腺泡
②mucous acinus	②黏液性腺泡
③interlobular duct	③小叶间导管

4.Pancreas

The surface of pancreas is covered with a connective tissue capsule, which extends into pancreas parenchyma and divides it into a few lobules with both exocrine and endocrine portions (Fig. 11-4).

Exocrine portion is composed of acini and ducts. All pancreas acini are serous, with round nucleus located near the base and perinuclear stained stronger basophilic. Centroacinar cells can be seen at the center of pancreas acini, where intercalated duct inserted, with oval nucleus, less cytoplasm and light stain. Pancreas intercalated duct has a narrower diameter, small lumen and light stain cytoplasm, with a simple layer of flat cells gradually changing to cuboidal epithelium (Fig. 11-5). The intralobular duct (without basal striations) of the pancreas connect with intercalated duct. Interlobular ducts are separated by interlobular septa, with simple columnar epithelium.

As compared with exocrine portion, endocrine portion of the pancreas is stained light pale, and called pancreas islets or islets of Langerhans, with groups of varied-size cells arranged in lumps and cords and abundant fenestrated capillaries among them (Fig. 11-6). Pancreas islets com-

4. 胰腺

胰腺表面有结缔组织被膜包裹，结缔组织伸入胰腺实质中将其分成若干小叶，小叶内既有内分泌部又有外分泌部（图11-4）。

外分泌部由腺泡和导管组成，胰腺的腺泡均为浆液性腺泡，浆液性腺细胞的核圆，近基底面，胞核周染色嗜碱性较强。胰腺腺泡中央可见泡心细胞，它是闰管插入腺泡的部分，泡心细胞核呈椭圆形，胞质少、染色浅淡。胰腺的闰管管径细、管腔小，胞质染色浅，形态从扁平逐渐向立方形过渡（图11-5）。与闰管相连的是小叶内导管，胰腺无纹状管。小叶间导管分布于小叶间隔中，上皮均为单层柱状上皮。

与外分泌部相比，内分泌部染色浅淡，称为胰岛。胰岛大小不等，细胞数量不一，排列成团索状，细胞间有丰富的毛细血管走行（图11-6）。胰岛由A细胞、B细胞和D细胞等组成，但在HE染色下无法区分，需要用特殊染色方

pose of A cells, B cells and D cells, and so on, which can not be distinguished in H.E. stain, and should be done by special stains. With AZAN stain (Fig. 11-7A), A cell is larger in size and with red cytoplasm, peripherally located surrounding the islets. B cell is smaller in size and with pink cytoplasm. With somatostatin-immunohistochemical stain, scattered D cells less in number in pancreas islets can be observed (Fig. 11-7B). B cells secreting insulin is the most numerous in pancreas islets, stained purplish-blue with histochemical stain. Number of B cells in pancreas islets and secretory granules in its cytoplasm in diabetic mouse (Fig. 11-8B) are apparently less than those in normal mouse (Fig. 11-8A).

法区分各类细胞。卡红-苯胺蓝（AZAN）染色中（图 11-7A），A细胞胞体较大，胞质被染成红色，多分布在胰岛的周边。B细胞胞体较小，胞质染色浅淡。利用抗生长抑素抗体-免疫组化方式染色，可观察D细胞的分布情况（图 11-7B），D细胞数量较少，在胰岛中散在分布。B细胞是胰岛中数量最多的细胞，分泌胰岛素。通过组化方式染色可见，被染成蓝紫色的细胞为B细胞。糖尿病小鼠的胰岛中（图 11-8B），B细胞的数量和胞质内的分泌颗粒数量明显比正常小鼠少（图 11-8A）。

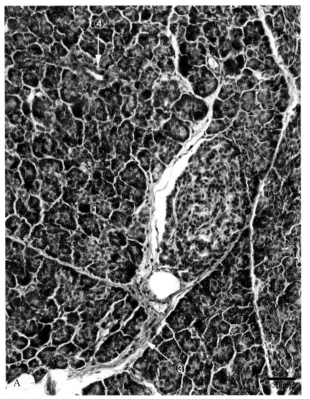
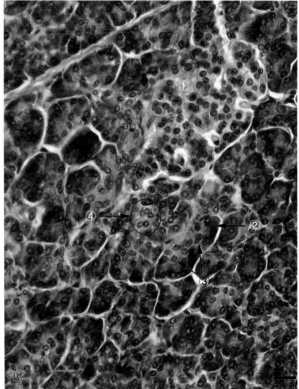

Fig. 11-4   Pancreas, by H.E. stain (slide No. DG4)
图 11-4　胰腺，HE 染色（切片 No. DG4）

A.Under low power objective
①exocrine portion of the pancreas
②endocrine portion of the pancreas
③interlobular septa
④intralobular duct
B.Under high power objective
①pancreas islet
②serous acinus
③centroacinar cells
④intercalated duct

A.低倍镜
①外分泌部
②内分泌部
③小叶间隔
④小叶内导管
B.高倍镜
①胰岛
②浆液性腺泡
③泡心细胞
④闰管

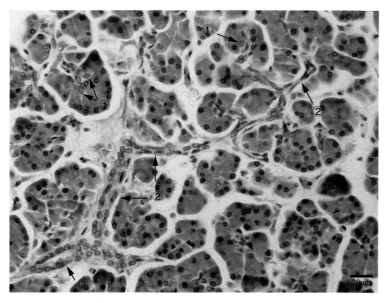

Fig. 11-5   Centroacinar cells and intercalated ducts of pancreas, by H.E.
stain (demonstration slide)

图11-5   胰腺，泡心细胞和闰管，HE染色（示教切片）

①centroacinar cells   ①泡心细胞
②intercalated duct   ②闰管

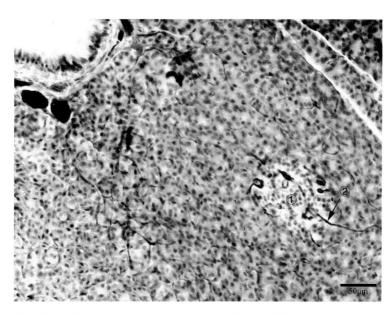

Fig. 11-6   Blood vessels in pancreas islet, from rabbit, by blood vessels
injection (demonstration slide)

图11-6   胰岛血管分布，兔，血管注射（示教切片）

①pancreas islet   ①胰岛
②capillary   ②毛细血管

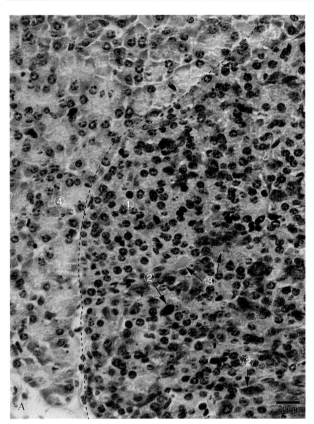

Fig. 11-7   Endocrine cells in pancrea islet

图 11-7   胰岛的细胞构成

A.Pancreas, from rabbit, by AZAN stain (demonstration slide)

①pancreas islet

②A cell

③capillary

④exocrine portion of pancreas

B.Pancreas, immunohistochemistry stain of somatostatin

(demonstration slide)

①pancreas islet

②D cell

A.胰腺，兔，卡红－苯胺蓝染色（示教切片）

①胰岛

②A 细胞

③毛细血管

④外分泌部

B.胰腺，生长抑素免疫组化染色（示教切片）

①胰岛

②D 细胞

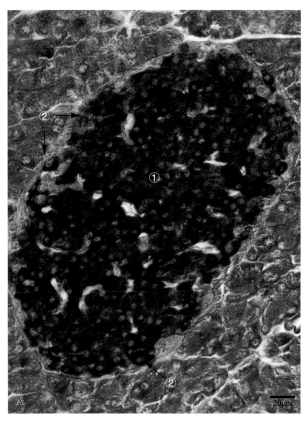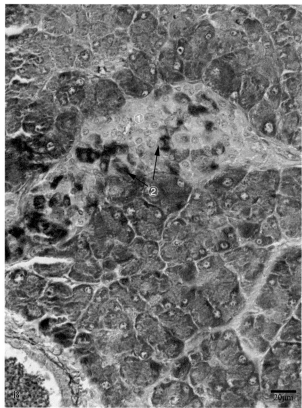

Fig. 11-8　B cells of pancreas islet, pancreas from mouse, by histochemical stain (demonstration slide)

图 11-8　胰岛B细胞，小鼠胰腺，组化染色（示教切片）

A.Normal mouse	A. 正常小鼠
① pancreas islet	① 胰岛
② B cell	② B细胞
B.Diabetic mouse	B. 糖尿病小鼠
① pancreas islet	① 胰岛
② B cell	② B细胞

5.Liver

(1) Liver lobule

Under microscope with low power objective, observing the liver section in H.E. stain (slide No. DG5), liver lobule appears hexagonal in shape on the whole. But, boundaries of human liver lobules are not clearly demarcated because of less connective tissue (Fig. 11-9B). Interlobular connective tissue is so apparent in pig liver, with clear lobular demarcation (Fig. 11-9A). Portal triad can be seen in connective tissue at lobular margin, i.e., interlobular arterioles, interlobular venules and interlobular bile ducts, referred to as portal area. Central vein is located in the center of each lobule, with larger lumen, thinner wall and less connective tissue beneath endothelium. Rows of hepatocytes radiate outward from the central

5.肝脏

（1）肝小叶

用低倍镜观察HE染色的肝脏切片No. DG5，肝小叶大致呈六角形，以结缔组织分隔，人的肝小叶间结缔组织较少，小叶边界不清晰（图11-9B）。猪的肝小叶间结缔组织明显，小叶边界清晰（图11-9A）。小叶边缘的结缔组织中可见门管三联体：小叶间动脉、小叶间静脉、小叶间胆管，这个区域被称为门管区。小叶中央为中央静脉，管腔大，管壁很薄，内皮下方结缔组织少。肝细胞以中央静脉为中心，放射状排列形成肝索，相邻肝索之间为肝血窦。来自小叶间动脉、小叶间静脉的血液流入肝血窦，之后依次汇入中央静脉和小叶下静脉。小叶下静脉单独走行，最终汇入肝静

vein toward the periphery of lobules forming hepatic cords, with hepatic blood sinusoids adjacent to them. Blood from interlobular arterioles and interlobular venules flows into hepatic sinusoids and converging into central veins and sublobular veins successively. Sublobular vein progresses alone and finally converges into hepatic vein leaving from the liver.

Observe the liver section by H.E. stain under microscope with high magnification, hepatocyte appears larger in size, spherical nucleus at its center, occasionally with bi-nuclei, and stronger acidophilic cytoplasm (Fig. 11-9C). Glycogen conversed from glucose after meals is stored in hepatocytes, which can be stained purplish-red in color by PAS stain (Fig. 11-9D). Hepatic sinusoid is irregular cavities lined with endothelial cells, with Kupffer cells seen in it, which are macrophages with phagocytic ability in the liver, with acidophilic cytoplasm and irregular light stain nuclei. Using carmine or trypan blue injected into peritoneal cavity of rat and then the rat autopsied about one week later, dyes granules phagocytized can be seen in the cytoplasm of its Kupffer cells (Fig. 11-10A). Reticular fibers as support-

脉出肝。

高倍镜下观察肝HE染色切片（图11-9C），肝细胞较大，核圆居中，偶尔有双核，胞质嗜酸性较强。进食后葡萄糖可转化为糖原储存在肝细胞内，PAS染色法可将糖原染成紫红色（图11-9D）。肝血窦为内皮细胞围成的不规则腔隙，血窦内可见库普弗细胞。库普弗细胞胞质呈嗜酸性，核不规则、染色较浅。库普弗细胞为肝内的巨噬细胞，具有吞噬能力。将卡红或台盼蓝等染料多次注射入大鼠腹腔，一周左右处死大鼠，可在肝脏库普弗细胞胞质内观察到被吞噬的染料（图11-10A）。肝细胞与肝血窦之间存在窦周隙，网状纤维分布于其间，起支持作用。因网状纤维具有嗜银性，银染时可观察到该纤维分布情况（图11-10B）。

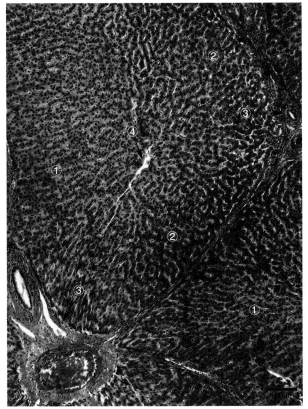
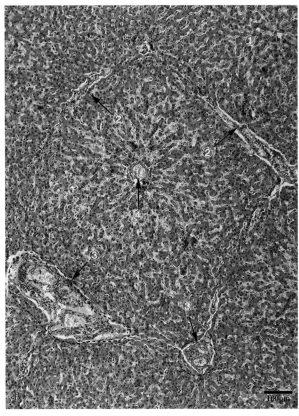

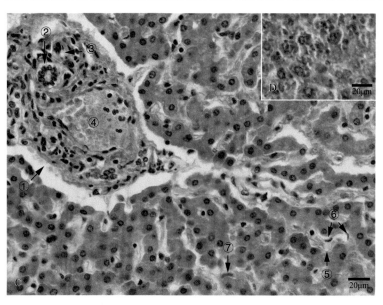

Fig. 11-9　Liver lobule, liver, by H.E. stain
图11-9　肝小叶，肝脏，HE染色

A.Pig hepatic lobules (demonstration slide)　　　　　　A.猪肝小叶（示教切片）

①liver lobule　　　　　　　　　　　　　　　　　①肝小叶

②septa of lobule　　　　　　　　　　　　　　　②小叶间隔

③portal area　　　　　　　　　　　　　　　　　③门管区

④central vein　　　　　　　　　　　　　　　　　④中央静脉

B.Human hepatic lobules (slide No. DG5)　　　　　　B.人肝小叶（切片 No. DG5）

①liver lobule　　　　　　　　　　　　　　　　　①肝小叶

②septa of lobule　　　　　　　　　　　　　　　②小叶间隔

③portal area　　　　　　　　　　　　　　　　　③门管区

④central vein　　　　　　　　　　　　　　　　　④中央静脉

C.Human hepatic lobules under high power objective (slide No.　C.人肝小叶高倍（切片 No. DG5）
DG5)

①portal area　　　　　　　　　　　　　　　　　①门管区

②interlobular bile ducts　　　　　　　　　　　　②小叶间胆管

③interlobular arteriole　　　　　　　　　　　　③小叶间动脉

④interlobular venule　　　　　　　　　　　　　④小叶间静脉

⑤hepatic sinusoid　　　　　　　　　　　　　　⑤肝血窦

⑥endothelial cell　　　　　　　　　　　　　　　⑥内皮细胞

⑦Kupffer cell　　　　　　　　　　　　　　　　⑦库普弗细胞

D.Glycogen granules in hepatocytes, by PAS stain (slide No. DG7)　D.肝细胞内糖原，肝脏，PAS染色（切片 No. DG7）

ing tissue scattered in the perisinusoidal space (Space
of Disse) between hepatocytes and hepatic sinusoids.
Reticular fiber is argyrophilic, so its distribution can be
seen with silver-impregnation method (Fig. 11-10B).

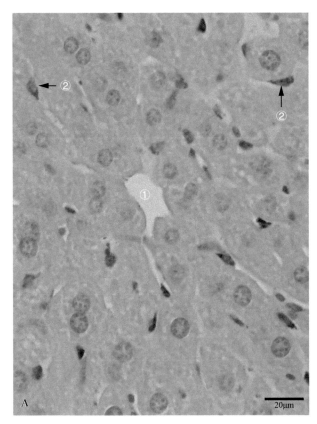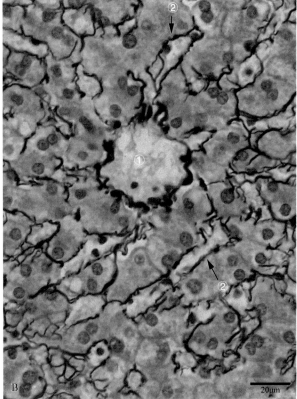

Fig. 11-10　Components of liver lobule
图 11-10　肝小叶组成成分

A.Kupffer cells, from rat, by carmine injection (slide No. DG6)

①central vein

②Kupffer cells

B.Reticular fibers, from guinea pig, by AgNO₃+azocarmine stain (demonstration slide)

①central vein

②reticular fibers

A.库普弗细胞，大鼠，卡红注射（切片 No. DG6）

①中央静脉

②库普弗细胞

B.网状纤维，豚鼠，硝酸银、偶氮卡红染色（示教切片）

①中央静脉

②网状纤维

(2) Bile transporting system

Bile synthesized by hepatocytes secretes into bile canaliculus, which formed by the inward concave surface of two adherent hepatocytes and cannot be observed in H.E. stain, and appears black in color by silver stain among hepatocytes (Fig. 11-11A). Hering canal (or intralobular bile canal) connecting with bile canaliculus is composed of single layer of cuboidal cholangiocytes, with less cytoplasm and light stain nucleus, scattered among hepatocytes adjacent to portal area and connected with interlobular bile ductules (Fig. 11-11B).

（2）胆汁运输管道

胆汁由肝细胞合成后排入胆小管，胆小管为相邻肝细胞胞膜向内凹陷形成，HE染色无法观察，银染时肝细胞间黑色的细管即为胆小管（图11-11A）。与胆小管相连的为Hering管（小叶内胆管），由单层立方的胆管上皮细胞围成，胞质少，染色浅淡，分布在肝细胞间，靠近门管区（图11-11B）。Hering管汇入门管区的小叶间胆管。

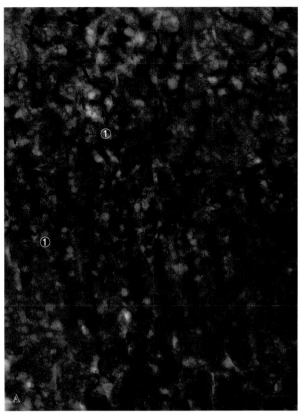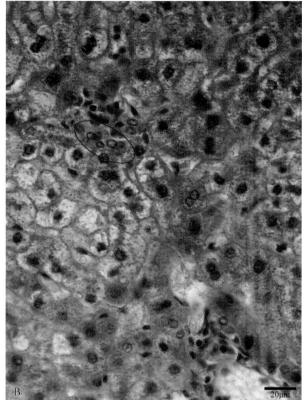

Fig. 11-11　Bile transporting system
图 11-11　胆汁运输管道

A.Liver biliary canaliculi, liver, from guinea pig, by AgNO₃ stain (slide No. DG8)

①biliary canaliculi

B.Hering canal, liver, from human, by H.E. stain (demonstration slide)

A.胆小管，肝，豚鼠，银染（切片No. DG8）

①胆小管

B.肝Hering管（小叶内胆管），人肝，HE染色（示教切片）

6.Gallbladder

Gallbladder, a hollow organ resembling a sack, mainly plays a role of bile condensation and storage. Its wall can be divided into three layers: mucosa, muscularis and adventitia. Mucosa includes epithelium and lamina propria, with the former composed of a simple columnar epithelia, and the mucosa extending into the lumen throwing up mucosal folds. Muscular layer is thin, with smooth muscle fiber arranged in bundles and interwoven with connective tissue. Except the part adjacent to liver composed of fibrosa, the remainder is covered with a layer of mesothelium, referred to serosa (Fig. 11-12).

6.胆囊

胆囊为中空性器官，主要起浓缩、储存胆汁的作用，管壁分3层：黏膜层、肌层和外膜层。黏膜包括上皮和固有层，上皮为单层柱状上皮，固有层较薄，黏膜伸向管腔形成皱襞。肌层较薄，肌纤维排列成束与结缔组织交织在一起。外膜层与肝脏相邻一侧为纤维膜，其余部分有一层间皮覆盖，为浆膜（图11-12）。

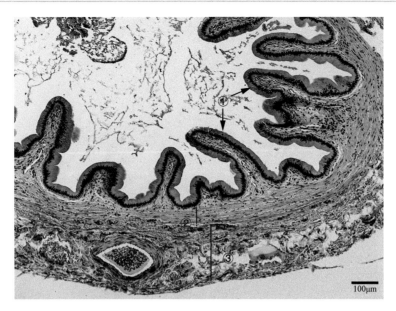

100μm

Fig. 11-12　Gallbladder, by H.E. stain (slide No. DG9)
图 11-12　胆囊，HE 染色（切片 No. DG9）

① mucosal folds　　　　　　①黏膜皱襞
② muscular layer　　　　　　②肌层
③ serosa　　　　　　　　　　③浆膜

Questions

1. How to distinguish parotid, submandibular gland, sublingual gland and pancreas?

2. How to distinguish gallbladder from the other tubular viscus, such as oviduct, small intestine, etc.?

问题

1.如何区分腮腺、下颌下腺、舌下腺和胰腺？

2.如何区分胆囊与其他中空性脏器，如输卵管、小肠等？

Chapter 12　DIGESTIVE TRACT

第十二章　消　化　管

Teaching and Learning Objectives

- To identify structures of four layers of the digestive tract wall: mucosa, submucosa, muscularis and adventitia, and to identify nerve plexus in submucosa and muscularis.
- To distinguish varied parts of the digestive tracts: esophagus, stomach, duodenum, jejunum, ileum, appendix and colon.
- To identify esophagus and describe characteristics of esophageal wall, such as those of esophageal epithelia, esophageal gland.
- To distinguish cardiac from fundus and pylorus of the stomach, to identify gastric gland of fundus, and to identify the surface mucous cells, chief cells and parietal cells, etc.
- To identify characteristic structures of small intestine, such as intestinal villi, crypts of Lieberkühn, central lacteal, and so on.To identify the characteristic cells of the small intestinal epithelia, such as Paneth cells, absorptive cells, goblet cells, etc. To distinguish the three parts of the small intestine, i.e., duodenum, jejunum and ileum, and to identify characteristic structure of its varied parts, such as duodenal gland, aggregate lymphoid nodules of ileum, etc.
- To identify characteristic structure of large intestine, and to distinguish appendix from colon.
- To distinguish gastroesophageal junction from gastroduodenal junction.

教学目标

- 辨认消化管管壁的4层结构，黏膜层、黏膜下层、肌层、外膜层；辨认黏膜下神经丛和肌间神经丛。
- 区分消化管各个部分：食管、胃、十二指肠、空肠、回肠、阑尾、结肠。
- 辨认食管，描述食管管壁的特点，如食管上皮、食管腺。
- 区分胃贲门、胃体和幽门，辨认胃小凹、胃底腺，辨认表面黏液细胞、胃底腺主细胞、壁细胞等。
- 辨认小肠的特征性结构，如小肠绒毛、小肠隐窝、中央乳糜管等，辨认小肠上皮的特征细胞，如潘氏细胞、小肠吸收细胞、杯状细胞等。区分小肠的3个部分，十二指肠、空肠、回肠，辨认各部分特征性的结构，如十二指肠腺、回肠集合淋巴小结等。
- 辨认大肠的特征性结构，区分阑尾、结肠。
- 区分食管－胃连接和胃－十二指肠连接。

In learning components of the alimentary tract, observe the following structures:

在学习消化管切片的时候注意观察以下结构：

1) mucosa ⎰ epithelium
⎱ lamina propria
⎱ muscularis mucosa

2) submucosa

3) muscularis

4) serosa or adventitia

Note particularly the characteristics of epithelia and mucosal glands in each case, which will help you distinguish varied segments of the digestive tract.

1.Tongue

See Chapter 10 Skin and Tongue.

2.Esophagus

Observing esophagus in slide No. DT 4 under microscope with low power objective, note to distinguish varied structure of four layers of the esophagus: mucosa, submucosa, muscularis and adventitia. Both mucosa and submucosa layers protrude to the lumen forming longitudinal folds. Esophageal lumen is lined with nonkeratinized stratified squamous epithelium, with the lamina propria underneath composed of loose connective tissue. The lamina propria and submucosa both composed of connective tissue are separated by the muscularis mucosae. Different from that in other digestive organs, esophageal muscularis mucosae only has one longitudinal layer of smooth muscle, the thicker of muscularis mucosae as it more approaching to the cardia (demonstration slide: gastroesophageal junction). Esophageal glands composed of mucous acini can be seen in the submucosa, with its secretion excreted to esophageal lumen via the ducts, involving in moisture and lubrication of the ingested food. Epithelia of the duct gradually transit to stratified epithelia from simple cuboidal epithelium, and immune cells, such as lymphocytes, etc., around the gland duct can be seen (Fig. 12-1). Muscularis is very thick, including inner circular muscle layer and outer longitudinal muscle layer. Types of muscles seen under microscope depend on the sites of sampling in tissue preparation. If sampled from the upper one-third of the esophagus, skeletal muscle can be seen, if sampled from the lower one-third, smooth muscle can be seen, and if sampled from the middle one-third, skeletal muscle mixed with smooth muscles can be seen. Sampling site can be judged simply by the types of

1）黏膜 ⎰ 上皮
⎱ 固有层
⎱ 黏膜肌层

2）黏膜下层

3）肌层

4）浆膜或纤维膜

注意观察每个器官上皮和黏膜腺的特征，这将有助于区分消化管的各部分结构。

1.舌

详见第十章：皮肤和舌。

2.食管

低倍镜下观察食管切片No. DT4，注意区分管壁的4层结构，黏膜层、黏膜下层、肌层和外膜层，黏膜层和黏膜下层共同向管壁隆起形成纵行皱襞。覆盖食管管腔的上皮是未角化的复层扁平上皮，其下方是由疏松结缔组织构成的固有层，黏膜肌层将均由结缔组织构成的固有层和黏膜下层分隔开。与消化管其他器官的黏膜肌层不同，食管的黏膜肌层只有一层纵向走行的平滑肌，而且越靠近胃贲门，黏膜肌层越厚（示教切片：食管胃交界）。黏膜下层中可见由黏液性腺泡构成的食管腺，其分泌物通过导管排入食管管腔，参与食物润滑。导管上皮从单层立方逐渐过渡到复层，导管周围常见淋巴细胞等免疫细胞分布（图12-1）。食管肌层很厚，包括内环、外纵2层，肌肉类型随取材部位不同而不同，如果从食管上1/3取材则为骨骼肌，下1/3取材为平滑肌，中间1/3为骨骼肌和平滑肌混合。可根据自己切片上肌层的肌肉类型，简单判断取材部位。两个肌层间的结缔组织中有肌间神经丛分布，黏膜下层中有黏膜下神经丛分布，分别用于调节肌层和黏膜肌层肌肉的运动。食管最外层为纤维膜，其与周围的结缔组织间无明显分界。

muscles seen in the slide. Myenteric nerve plexus spreads in the connective tissue between two muscular layers, and submucosa nerve plexus spreads in the submucosa, which regulate the muscular movement of the muscularis and muscularis mucosae, respectively. The outermost layer of esophagus is fibrosa, without clear demarcation with connective tissue around it.

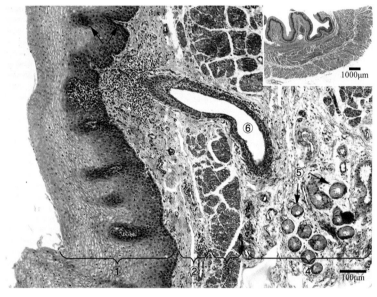

Fig. 12-1　Esophagus, by H.E. stain (slide No. DT4)

图12-1　食管，HE染色（切片No. DT4）

①stratified squamous epithelium	①复层扁平上皮
②lamina propria	②固有层
③muscularis mucosae	③黏膜肌层
④submucosa	④黏膜下层
⑤mucous acini of eso-phageal gland	⑤食管腺黏液性腺泡
⑥duct of esophageal gland	⑥食管腺导管
⑦papilla of connective tissue	⑦结缔组织乳头
Illustration (inserted): esophagus under low power objective	图中图：食管低倍照片

1000μm

100μm

3.Stomach

(1) Fundus

The surface of stomach covers a layer of columnar, mucous secreting cells-the surface mucous cells. At intervals the epithelium dips downward forming the gastric pits. Numerous mucosal glands distributed in lamina propria open into the bases of the gastric pits (Fig. 12-2, Fig. 12-3).

Histological structure of the mucosal gland in fundus is similar to that of in the body of stomach, called gastric gland. The gastric gland is composed with varied cells and its parietal cells can be easily distinguished from chief cells in H.E. stain. Parietal cells distribute close to the upper part of gastric gland, larger in size, with round and centrally-located nuclei and stronger acidophilic cytoplasm. Chief (or zymogenic) cells mostly distribute in the lower part of gastric gland, numerous in quantity, with round nuclei near the base of cells and stronger basophilic cytoplasm. Enteroendocrine cells are not easily identified in H.E. stain. There are mucous

3.胃

（1）胃底

覆盖在胃表面的为单层柱状上皮，均由表面黏液细胞组成，细胞胞质染色浅淡。上皮向下凹陷形成胃小凹，胃底腺（黏膜腺）开口在胃小凹处（图12-2，图12-3）。

分布在胃底和胃体的黏膜腺结构相似，均称为胃底腺。胃底腺构成细胞种类多，HE染色时壁细胞和主细胞容易分辨。壁细胞分布靠近胃底腺的上半部分，细胞大，核圆居中，胞质强嗜酸性。主细胞多分布于胃底腺下半部分，数量多，核圆近基底部，核周的胞质嗜碱性较强。内分泌细胞在HE染色时不易辨认。胃底腺颈部（近胃小凹处）有颈黏液细胞分布，细胞核不规则，胞质染色浅，HE染色时不易辨认。

neck cells in the neck of gastric gland (near gastric pit), with irregular nuclei and light-stain cytoplasm, and can not easily be identified in H.E. stain.

Muscularis externa of the stomach is composed with smooth muscle, and can be divided into three layers, i.e., inner oblique, middle circular and outer longitudinal muscle layers, but not all these three layers can be identified apparently. The outer layer of the stomach is serosa.

胃的肌层均由平滑肌构成，分为内斜、中环、外纵3层，但这3层结构并不是在胃的所有区域都能清晰辨认。胃的外膜为浆膜。

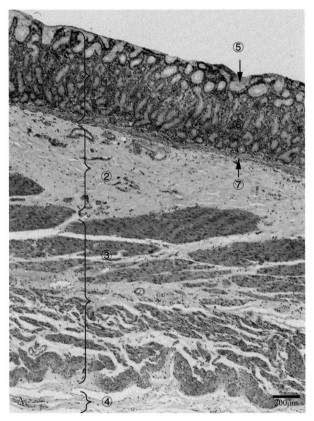
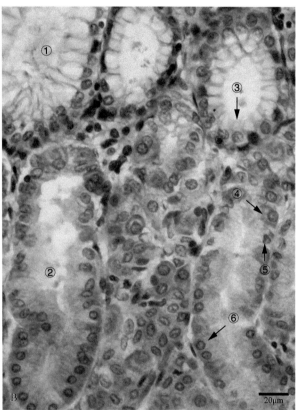

Fig. 12-2   Gastric fundus, from human, by H.E. stain (slide No. DT5)
图 12-2   胃底，人，HE染色（切片No. DT5）

A.Structure of stomach fundus
①mucosa
②submucosa
③muscularis externa
④serosa
⑤gastric pits
⑥gastric glands
⑦muscularis mucosae
B.Gastric pit and gastric gland
①gastric pit
②gastric gland
③surface mucous cells
④parietal cells
⑤mucous neck cells
⑥chief cells

A. 胃底结构
①黏膜层
②黏膜下层
③肌层
④浆膜层
⑤胃小凹
⑥胃底腺
⑦黏膜肌层
B. 胃小凹和胃底腺
①胃小凹
②胃底腺
③表面黏液细胞
④壁细胞
⑤颈黏液细胞
⑥主细胞

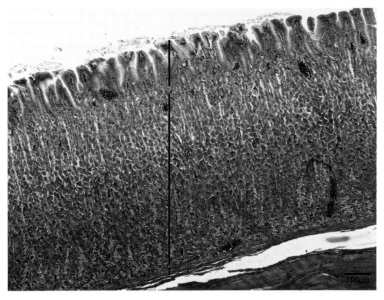

Fig. 12-3　Fundus, from rabbit, by H.E. stain (slide No. DT6)

图12-3　胃底，兔，HE染色（切片No. DT6）

① gastric pits　　　　　　　　　　　　① 胃小凹
② gastric glands　　　　　　　　　　　② 胃底腺
③ muscularis mucosae　　　　　　　　③ 黏膜肌层

(2) Gastro-esophageal junction and gastro-duodenal junction

Observe structures of the mucosa in gastric cardia and pylorus in the demonstration slide of gastro-esophageal junction (Fig. 12-4) and gastro-duodenal junction (Fig. 12-5). The gastric pit is shallower in the cardia, and deeper in the pylorus as depth as a half of thickness of the mucosa. Both cardiac gland and pyloric gland are mucous in nature and their secretions provide better protection for the mucosa.

Observe the demonstration slides of gastro-esophageal junction and gastro-duodenal junction, and think about what are the structural characteristics of mucosa (epithelium, lamina propria muscularis mucosae), submucosa, muscularis externa and adventitia in the esophagus, gastric cardia, pylorus and duodenum, which can help you (to) distinguish these organs?

（2）食管-胃连接和胃-十二指肠连接

在食管-胃连接示教切片（图12-4）和胃-十二指肠连接示教切片（图12-5）观察胃贲门和幽门的黏膜层结构。胃小凹在贲门处较浅，但在幽门处可深达黏膜层的二分之一。贲门腺和幽门腺均为黏液腺，其分泌物对黏膜起到较好的保护作用。

观察食管-胃连接和胃-十二指肠连接示教切片，思考食管、胃贲门、胃幽门、十二指肠在黏膜层（上皮、固有层黏膜肌层）、黏膜下层、肌层、外膜层都有什么特征性结构，如何帮助我们去辨别这些器官？

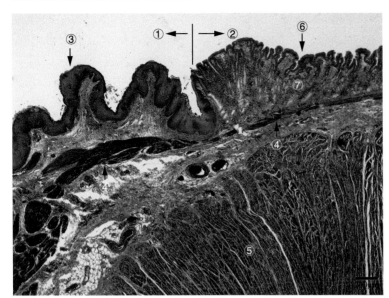

Fig. 12-4   Gastro-esophageal junction, from cat, by H.E. stain (demonstration slide)

图12-4   食管-胃贲门连接，猫，HE染色（示教切片）

① esophagus   ①食管
② cardia   ②贲门
③ stratified squamous epithelium   ③复层扁平上皮
④ muscularis mucosae   ④黏膜肌层
⑤ muscularis   ⑤肌层
⑥ gastric pits   ⑥胃小凹
⑦ cardiac glands   ⑦贲门腺

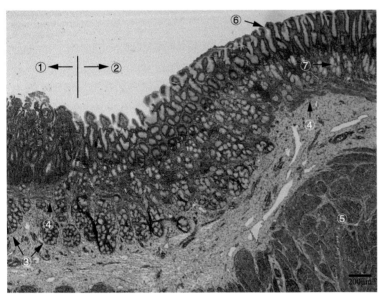

Fig. 12-5   Gastro-duodenal junction, by H.E. stain (demonstration slide)

图12-5   胃十二指肠连接，HE染色（示教切片）

① duodenum   ①十二指肠
② pylorus   ②胃幽门
③ duodenal gland   ③十二指肠腺
④ muscularis mucosae   ④黏膜肌层
⑤ pyloric sphincter   ⑤幽门括约肌
⑥ gastric pit   ⑥胃小凹
⑦ pyloric gland   ⑦幽门腺

4. Small intestine

(1) Jejunum

This is a longitudinal section of jejunum with H.E. stain (slide No. DT8). The largest protruding structure that can be seen by naked eyes is called plica circulares, and the structure formed by the mucosa and submucosa protruding into jejunal lumen (Fig. 12-6A). Finger-like structure protruding into intestinal lumen from plica circulares is called intestinal villus, which is composed of epithelia and lamina propria. Intestinal gland (or crypt of Lieberkuhn) is formed by epithelia invaginated towards the lamina propria, with its epithelia continuing to that of intestinal villus mutually. Small intestine

4. 小肠

（1）空肠

切片No. DT8是空肠纵切的HE染色切片，肉眼可见最大一级的突起为环形皱襞，光镜下可见其为黏膜层和黏膜下层共同向管腔突起形成的结构（图12-6A）。黏膜皱襞上向管腔突起的指状结构为小肠绒毛，它是由上皮和固有层共同形成的。上皮向固有层方向凹陷形成小肠腺，小肠腺与小肠绒毛的上皮相互延续。小肠绒毛是小肠的特征性结构，绒毛轴心的结缔组织中可见管腔大、壁薄的中央乳糜管，它是小肠的吸收细胞吸收脂类后的运输通道。黏膜下层有丰富的血管和神经分布（图12-6B），注意

is characterized by its intestinal villi. Central lacteal (or lymphatic capillary) with bigger lumen and thinner wall can be seen in the connective tissue as the center of intestinal villus, a passage that lipids absorbed by small intestine transported through. Submucosa contains abundant blood vessels and nerves (Fig. 12-6B). Note to find nerve plexus in the submucosa, and observe whether there is solitary lymphoid nodule and diffused lymphoid tissue there. Find myenteric nerve plexus in the inner circular and outer longitudinal muscle layers and observe nerve fibers and neuron in the plexus. Think about the orientation of smooth muscle arranged in the inner circular and outer longitudinal muscle layers, as sampling for preparation of transverse and longitudinal sections. The outer layer of the jejunum is serosa.

Under microscope with high power objective, epithelium of small intestine is composed of simple columnar cells, including absorptive cells, goblet cells, Paneth cells, enteroendocrine cells, stem cells, etc (Fig. 12-7A). Absorptive cells are the major cells in intestinal epithelium, with striated border seen at their apexes. Paneth cells locate at the base of intestinal gland, with round nuclei, containing lots of acidophilic secretory granules at their apexes (Fig. 12-7C). If secretory granules of the cells are dissolved in tissue preparation, their apical cytoplasm is vacuolated. Paneth cells can be distinguished from goblet cells by the shape of cells and their nuclei, the latter appearing dark-stained triangular nuclei and wine-cup in shape. Enteroendocrine cells can not be recognized in H.E. stain, and can be well done by silver salts impregnation stain, based on enteroendocrine cells containing argentaffin granules (Fig. 12-7B). Note the location of these dark brown granules in the cells. Think about why they are called basal granular cells. Mitotic cells can be seen in the lower part of intestinal gland.

寻找黏膜下神经丛，观察黏膜下层是否有孤立淋巴小结和弥散淋巴组织存在？在内环和外纵肌层之间寻找肌间神经丛，观察神经丛内的神经纤维和神经元细胞。思考空肠纵切和横切取材时，内环层和外纵层的平滑肌的切面方向。空肠的外膜层是浆膜。

高倍镜下可见小肠的上皮为单层柱状上皮，由吸收细胞、杯状细胞、潘氏细胞、内分泌细胞和干细胞等组成（图12-7A）。吸收细胞是小肠上皮中主要的细胞，其顶面可见纹状缘。潘氏细胞分布于小肠腺的基底部，细胞核圆，细胞顶部有大量嗜酸性的分泌颗粒（图12-7C），分泌颗粒如果在制片过程中被溶解，则细胞顶面成空泡状。此时可根据细胞和细胞核的形状区分潘氏细胞和杯状细胞（后者，细胞高脚杯状、核三角形、深染）。内分泌细胞HE染色不易区分，通过银染的方法可较好识别胞质内含嗜银颗粒的内分泌细胞（图12-7B），注意这些棕黑色颗粒在细胞内的位置，想想它们为什么叫作基底颗粒细胞？小肠腺的下半部分可见到正在分裂的细胞。

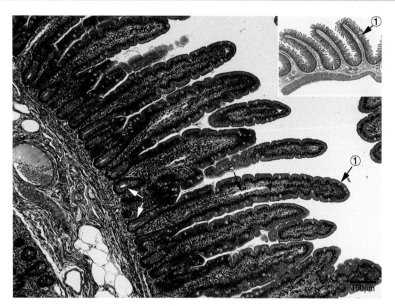

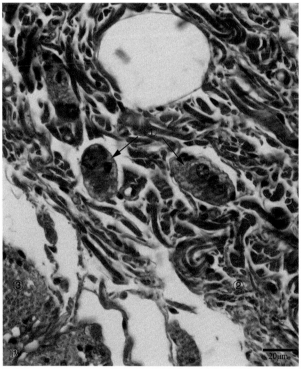

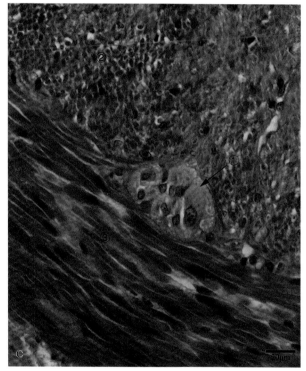

Fig. 12-6 Jejunum, by H.E. stain (slide No. DT8)
图12-6 空肠，HE染色（切片No. DT8）

A.Mucosa and submucosa of jejunum
①intestinal villus
②central lacteal
③intestinal glands
④submucosa
Illustration (inserted) : Jejunum, under low power objective
①plicae circulares
B.Submucosa
①submucosa nerve plexus
②submucosa
③muscularis
C.Muscularis
①myenteric nerve plexus
②inner circular layer of muscularis
③outer longitudinal layer of muscularis

A.空肠黏膜和黏膜下层
①小肠绒毛
②中央乳糜管
③小肠腺
④黏膜下层
图中图：空肠低倍
①环形皱襞
B.黏膜下层
①黏膜下神经丛
②黏膜下层
③肌层
C.肌层
①肌间神经丛
②肌层－内环层
③肌层－外纵层

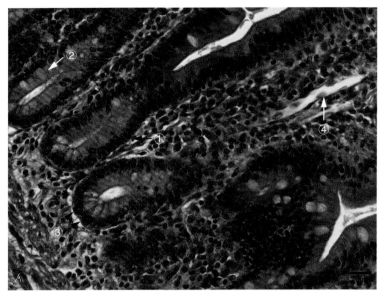

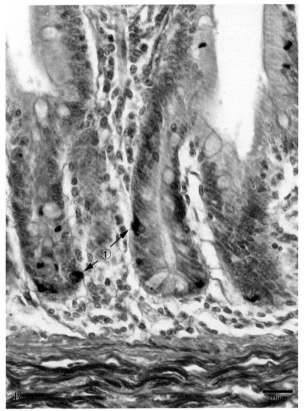

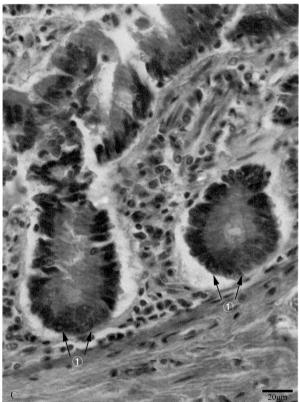

Fig. 12-7　Epithelial cells of the small intestine
图 12-7　小肠上皮细胞

A.Jejunum, under high power objective, by H.E. stain (slide No. DT8)

①absorptive cells

②goblet cells

③Paneth cells

④central lacteal

B.Argentaffin cells, by AgNO₃ stain (slide No. DT12)

①enteroendocrine cells (argentaffin cell, basal granular cells)

C.Paneth cells, from mouse, by H.E. stain (demonstration slide)

①Paneth cells

A.空肠高倍，HE 染色（切片 No. DT8）

①吸收细胞

②杯状细胞

③潘氏细胞

④中央乳糜管

B.嗜银细胞，银染（切片 No. DT12）

①内分泌细胞（嗜银细胞，基底颗粒细胞）

C.潘氏细胞，小鼠，HE 染色（示教切片）

①潘氏细胞

(2) Duodenum

Duodenal gland in the submucosa is an identification marker for the duodenum. Duodenal gland is mucous in nature for human (Fig. 12-5), but serous for cat (Fig. 12-8).

（2）十二指肠

黏膜下层的十二指肠腺是十二指肠的识别标志，人的十二指肠腺为黏液腺（图12-5），但猫的为浆液腺（图12-8）。

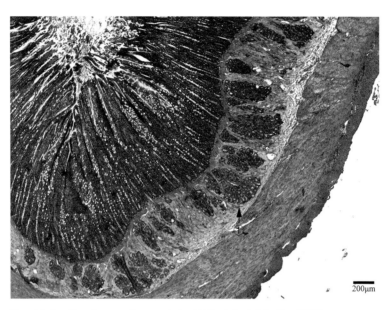

Fig. 12-8　Duodenum, from cat, by H.E. stain (slide No. DT7)
图12-8　十二指肠，猫，HE染色（切片No. DT7）

①duodenal gland (gland of Brunner)　　　①十二指肠腺

(3) Ileum

Aggregated lymphoid nodule is an identification marker for ileum, with lymphoid nodules aggregate together, known as Peyer patches, break through the muscularis mucosae and occupy the submucosa (Fig. 12-9). Note to observe difference among the epithelia of intestinal villi, intestinal gland, and that of the surface of lymphoid nodules. There are microfold cells (M cells) on surface epithelium of lymphoid nodule, which present antigens to lymphocytes and macrophages underneath and cannot be distinguished in H.E. stain, and only some lymphocytes can be found in the epithelium.

（3）回肠

集合淋巴小结是回肠的识别标志，淋巴小结聚集在一起，突破黏膜肌层占据黏膜下层（图12-9）。注意观察淋巴小结表面的上皮与小肠绒毛、小肠腺的上皮有什么差别？淋巴小结表面的上皮存在微皱褶细胞（M细胞），将抗原呈递给下方淋巴细胞和巨噬细胞等，该细胞在HE染色时无法辨认，仅在上皮中见到一些淋巴细胞分布。

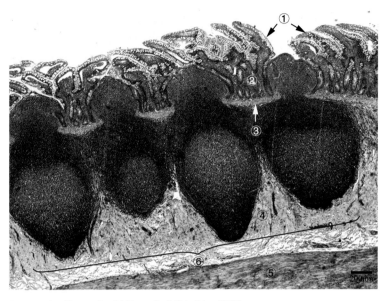

Fig. 12-9   Ileum, by H.E. stain (slide No. DT9)

图12-9   回肠，HE染色（切片No. DT9）

①intestinal villi

②intestinal gland

③muscularis mucosae

④submucosa

⑤muscularis

⑥aggregate lymphoid nodules (Peyer patches)

①小肠绒毛

②小肠腺

③黏膜肌层

④黏膜下层

⑤肌层

⑥集合淋巴小结

5.Large intestine

(1) Colon

Surface of the colon has no villus protruding into the lumen. Large intestine gland in lamina propria is lined with simple columnar epithelium, with numerous goblet cells among the absorptive cells. Adipocytes and isolated lymphoid nodules can be seen in the submucosa. The muscularis externa composed of inner circular and outer longitudinal smooth muscle layers (Fig. 12-10), with the latter thickened locally forming the teniae coli (Fig. 12-11).

5. 大肠

（1）结肠

结肠没有向管腔突起的肠绒毛结构，单层柱状上皮向固有层凹陷形成大肠腺，吸收细胞间有大量杯状细胞。黏膜下层可见脂肪细胞和孤立淋巴小结。肌层由内环、外纵2层平滑肌构成（图12-10），纵行肌局部可增厚成结肠带（图12-11）。

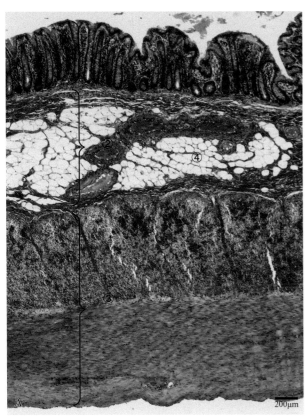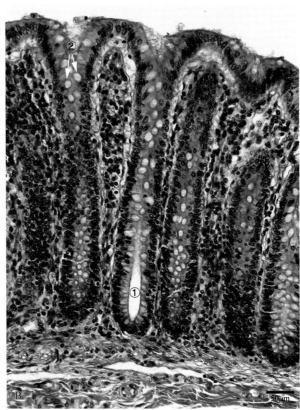

Fig. 12-10　Colon, by H.E. stain (slide No. DT10)

图12-10　结肠，HE染色（切片No. DT10）

A.Colon

①mucosa

②submucosa

③muscularis

④adipose tissue

B.Mucosa of colon

①large intestinal gland

②goblet cells

A.结肠

①黏膜层

②黏膜下层

③肌层

④脂肪组织

B.结肠黏膜层

①大肠腺

②杯状细胞

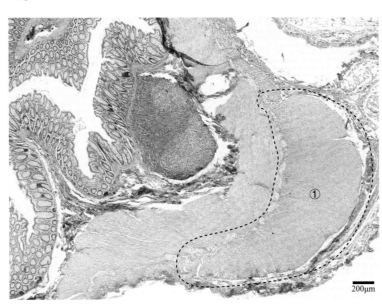

Fig. 12-11　Teniae coli, from monkey, by H.E. stain (demonstration slide)

图12-11　结肠带，猴，HE染色（示教切片）

①teniae coli　　　　　①结肠带

123

(2) Appendix

Appendix is characterized by a relatively small and narrow lumen, and fecalith (digestive residuals) can usually be seen in it. Large intestinal gland is shallow and less in number. Lots of diffused lymphoid tissues and nodules can be seen in the lamina propria, with most lymphoid nodules breaking through the muscularis mucosae and penetrating to the submucosa. Muscularis is composed of outer longitudinal and inner circular muscle layers, and the outermost layer is serosa (Fig. 12-12).

（2）阑尾

阑尾的管腔较小，常可见消化物残渣堆积。大肠腺较浅且数量较少，固有层可见大量弥散淋巴组织和淋巴小结，淋巴小结多突破黏膜肌层到达黏膜下层。黏膜下层较薄，肌层由内环、外纵2层构成，外膜为浆膜（图12-12）。

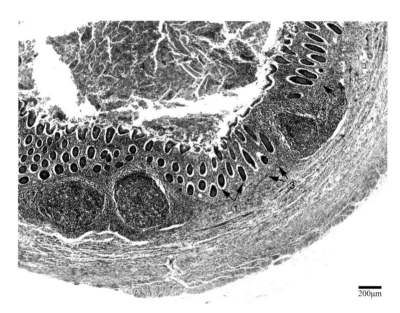

200μm

Fig. 12-12　Appendix, by H.E. stain (slide No. DT11)
图12-12　阑尾，HE染色（切片No. DT11）

①large intestinal gland
②lymphoid nodule
③muscularis mucosae
④fecalith

①大肠腺
②淋巴小结
③黏膜肌层
④粪石

Questions

1.How to distinguish varied parts of the digestive tract?

2.How to distinguish digestive tract organs from the other tubular organs?

问题

1.如何区分消化管的各个部分？

2.消化管各器官如何与其他管状器官区分？

Chapter 13　RESPIRATORY SYSTEM

第十三章　呼吸系统

Teaching and Learning Objectives

- To identify histological structure of nasal mucosa, and know morphological difference between the respiratory portion and the olfactory portion.
- To identify histological structure of trachea.
- To identify morphological features of varied branches of bronchial tree.
- To identify morphological features of type Ⅰ and type Ⅱ pulmonary cells.

教学目标

- 辨认鼻黏膜的组织学结构，区分呼吸部和嗅部的形态学差异。
- 辨认气管的组织学结构。
- 辨认支气管树各级分支的形态学特点。
- 辨认Ⅰ型肺泡细胞和Ⅱ型肺泡细胞的形态特点。

Respiratory system divided into two principal divisions: the conducting portion and the respiratory portion.

1.Nasal cavity

This is a coronal section through nasal septum. The lower part of nasal cavity is the respiratory portion, and its mucosa is lined with pseudostratified ciliated columnar epithelium with numerous goblet cells among it. Lamina propria is richly vascularized and has many serous and mucous glands, attached to the perichondrium of nasal septum. The olfactory portion locates in the roof of nasal cavity, and its olfactory epithelium is thick, pseudostratified columnar epithelium containing three types of cells. Olfactory cells are bipolar neurons with round nuclei and dendritic processes extending to the free surface of the epithelium, and axons penetrating the basement membrane and forming bundles of nerve fibers. Sustentacular (or supporting) cells are elongated columnar cells and basal cells are small conical cells with flat nuclei lying closer to the basement membrane . Serous glands present in lamina propria, and the deeper layer of lamina propria is periosteum of bony nasal septum (Fig. 13-1, Fig. 13-2).

呼吸系统主要分为两部分：导气部和呼吸部。

1.鼻腔

切片为通过鼻中隔的冠状切面。鼻腔下部是呼吸部，黏膜由假复层纤毛柱状上皮覆盖，内有大量杯状细胞，固有层中富含血管，内有浆液腺和黏液腺，固有层与鼻中隔的软骨膜直接相连。嗅部位于鼻腔的顶部，嗅上皮是高的假复层柱状上皮，包含3种细胞，嗅细胞是双极神经元，核圆，树突伸向游离面，轴突穿过基底膜形成神经束；支持细胞是高柱状细胞；基细胞是小的锥体形细胞，核扁平，靠近基底膜。浆液腺存在于固有层，固有层深层是骨性鼻中隔的骨膜（图13-1，图13-2）。

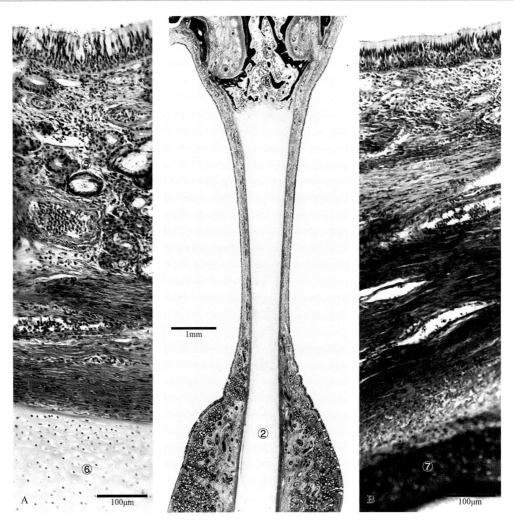

Fig. 13-1　Nasal septum, by azocarmine stain (slide No. Re1)

图13-1　鼻中隔，偶氮卡红染色（切片No. Re1）

A. Respiratory portion; B. Olfactory portion

① olfactory portion

② respiratory portion

③ pseudostratified ciliated columnar epithelium

④ pseudostratified columnar epithelium

⑤ lamina propria

⑥ (hyaline) cartilaginous nasal septum

⑦ bony nasal septum

A. 呼吸部；B. 嗅部

①嗅部

②呼吸部

③假复层纤毛柱状上皮

④假复层柱状上皮

⑤固有层

⑥（透明）软骨性鼻中隔

⑦骨性鼻中隔

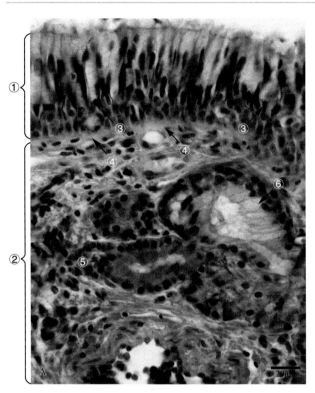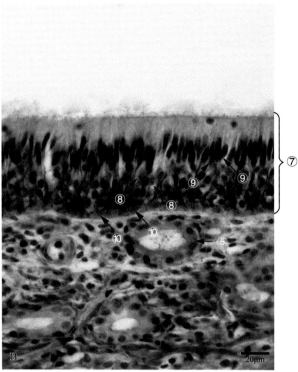

Fig. 13-2　Nasal septum, by azocarmine stain (slide No. Re1)
图 13-2　鼻中隔，偶氮卡红染色（切片 No. Re1）

A. Respiratory portion; B. Olfactory portion
① respiratory epithelium
② lamina propria
③ goblet cell
④ basement membrane
⑤ serous gland
⑥ mucous gland
⑦ olfactory epithelium
⑧ olfactory cell
⑨ supporting cell
⑩ basal cell

A. 呼吸部；B. 嗅部
① 呼吸上皮
② 固有层
③ 杯状细胞
④ 基膜
⑤ 浆液腺
⑥ 黏液腺
⑦ 嗅上皮
⑧ 嗅细胞
⑨ 支持细胞
⑩ 基细胞

2.Trachea

This is the cross section of trachea. Trachea is lined with typical respiratory mucosa, which is pseudostratified ciliated columnar epithelium with goblet cells and prominent basement membrane. Mixed tracheal gland lies principally in the submucosa, and its adventitia contains hyaline cartilage. Lymphocytes can frequently be seen in the wall of trachea (Fig. 13-3).

2.气管

切片为气管的横切面。气管由典型的呼吸黏膜覆盖，黏膜上皮是假复层纤毛柱状上皮，内有杯状细胞，基膜明显。混合性气管腺主要分布于黏膜下层，外膜层包含透明软骨。管壁中常见淋巴细胞（图 13-3）。

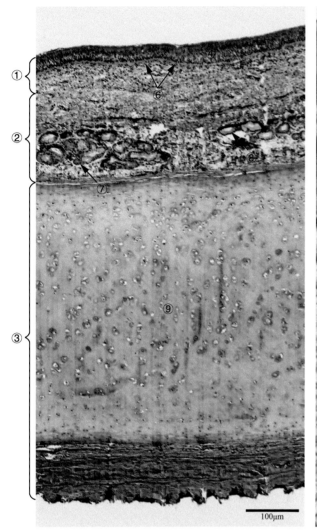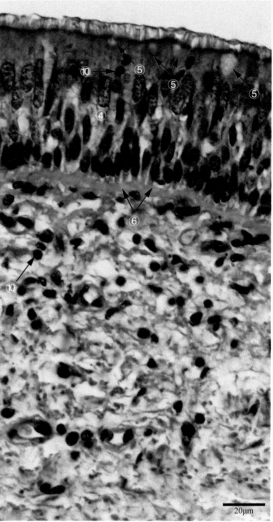

Fig. 13-3　Trachea, by H.E. stain (slide No. Re2)

图 13-3　气管，HE 染色（切片 No. Re2）

①mucosa

②submucosa

③adventitia

④pseudostratified ciliated columnar epithelium

⑤goblet cell

⑥basement membrane

⑦serous acinus

⑧mucous acinus

⑨hyaline cartilage

⑩lymphocyte

①黏膜

②黏膜下层

③外膜

④假复层纤毛柱状上皮

⑤杯状细胞

⑥基膜

⑦浆液腺泡

⑧黏液腺泡

⑨透明软骨

⑩淋巴细胞

3.Lung

Identify small bronchi, whose wall has a few small plaques of cartilage and mixed gland and whose lumen is lined with respiratory epithelium and intervened with some thin and discontinuous smooth muscle fibers between epithelium and

3.肺

辨认小支气管，管壁中有一些小的软骨片和混合腺，呼吸上皮覆盖管腔，上皮和软骨之间有一些薄而不连续的平滑肌纤维。随着分支，小支气管越变越小，杯状细胞消失，柱状

cartilage. As small bronchi become smaller and smaller with their branching, the goblet cells in epithelia disappear and the columnar epithelial cells lose their cilia gradually. The terminal bronchiole is covered with simple columnar or cuboidal epithelium, and its next-level respiratory bronchiole lined with simple cuboidal epithelium and alveolar openings. Branching further, next to respiratory bronchiole is alveolar duct with thinner and discontinuous wall, and lots of alveolar openings.

上皮失去纤毛。终末细支气管由单层柱状或立方上皮覆盖，其下一级为呼吸性细支气管，由单层立方上皮覆盖，上有肺泡开口；其再下一级分支为肺泡管，管壁变得不连续，有大量肺泡开口，相邻肺泡之间有薄层结缔组织构成的肺泡隔，肺泡隔末端有平滑肌细胞构成的结节状膨大（图13-4）。

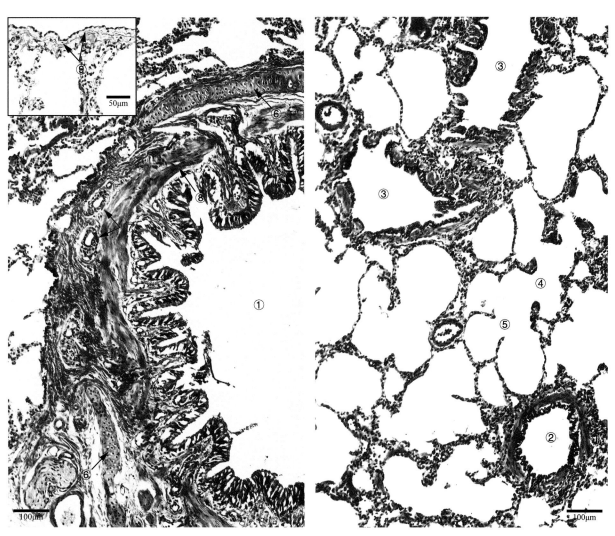

Fig. 13-4   Lung, by H.E. stain (slide No. Re3)
图13-4   肺，HE染色（切片No. Re3）

① small bronchus
② terminal bronchiole
③ respiratory bronchiole
④ alveolar duct
⑤ alveolar sac
⑥ hyaline cartilage
⑦ mixed gland
⑧ smooth muscle
⑨ mesothelium

①小支气管
②终末细支气管
③呼吸性细支气管
④肺泡管
⑤肺泡囊
⑥透明软骨
⑦混合腺
⑧平滑肌
⑨间皮

There are thinner alveolar septa of connective tissue between adjacent alveoli, with expanded nodular knobs composed of smooth muscle cells at their terminal (Fig. 13-4).

Observe structure of alveolar wall. Try to find an appropriate region in the slide, and to identify the following three types of cells:

Alveolar wall is mainly lined with flattened type Ⅰ pneumocytes (or type Ⅰ alveolar cells), with elongate nuclei and unclearly visible cytoplasm under light microscope. Capillary endothelium in the alveolar septum is also composed of simple squamous epithelium, with nuclei bulging into its lumen, but nuclei of type Ⅰ pneumocytes bulge into the alveolar space, distinguishing from each other in favorable regions of the section.

Type Ⅱ pneumocyte (or type Ⅱ alveolar cell) is cuboidal in shape, with round nuclei and abundant vacuolated, lightly stained cytoplasm, scattered solitarily or in cluster among type Ⅰ alveolar cells.

There are many alveolar macrophages (dust cells) within alveolar lumen or among connective tissue of the lung, containing lots of granules with oval nuclei (Fig. 13-5).

观察肺泡壁的结构，找一个合适的区域辨认以下3种类型的细胞：

肺泡壁主要由扁平的Ⅰ型肺泡细胞覆盖，核细长，胞质光镜下不清晰。肺泡隔中的毛细血管内皮也是单层扁平上皮，其核凸向血管腔，而Ⅰ型肺泡细胞核凸向肺泡腔，二者在切片适合的区域可以据此区分。

Ⅱ型肺泡细胞是立方形细胞，核圆形，胞质染色浅，呈泡沫样，单个或成群分布于Ⅰ型肺泡细胞之间。

在肺泡腔或者结缔组织中有很多含有颗粒的肺泡巨噬细胞（尘细胞），核呈卵圆形（图13-5）。

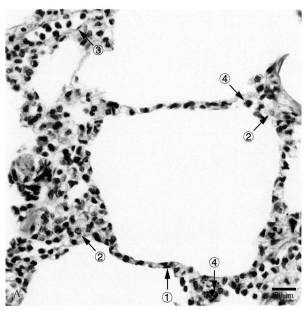
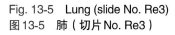
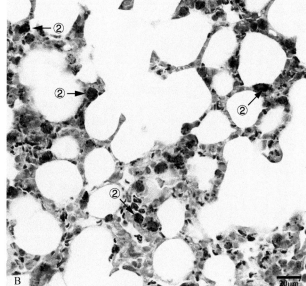

Fig. 13-5　Lung (slide No. Re3)
图 13-5　肺（切片 No. Re3）

A.by H.E. stain; B.by osmic acid stain
①type Ⅰ alveolar cell (or type Ⅰ pneumocytes)
②type Ⅱ alveolar cell (or type Ⅱ pneumocytes)
③endothelial cell
④alveolar macrophages (dust cells)

A.HE 染色；B.锇酸染色
①Ⅰ型肺泡细胞
②Ⅱ型肺泡细胞
③内皮细胞
④肺泡巨噬细胞（尘细胞）

4.Blood vessels of lung

Branches of the pulmonary arteries and veins conduct blood under relatively low pressure and, consequently, are thin-walled. Observe the extensive capillary plexus in the wall of the alveoli taken from a rat injected intravascularly with India ink (Fig. 13-6).

4.肺血管

肺动脉和肺静脉分支的血管内压力相对较低，所以管壁也较薄。仔细观察大鼠血管内注射印度墨水后显示的肺泡壁毛细血管丛（图13-6）。

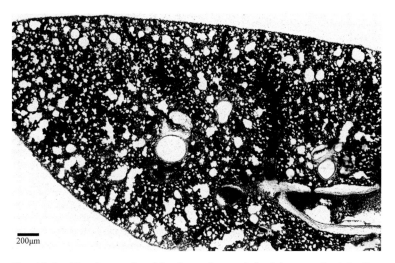

200μm

Fig. 13-6   Blood vessels of the lung, from rat, by intravascular injection with India ink (demonstration slide)
图13-6   肺血管，大鼠血管内印度墨水注射（示教切片）

Questions

How to distinguish the respiratory portion of nasal cavity from its olfactory portion in the light microscope?

问题

如何在光镜下区分鼻腔的呼吸部和嗅部？

Chapter 14 URINARY SYSTEM
第十四章 泌尿系统

Teaching and Learning Objectives

- To identify cortex and medulla in the kidney, as well as cortical labyrinth and medullary rays in renal cortex.
- To identify structure of renal corpuscle: vascular pole and tubular pole, glomerulus, Bowman's capsule and podocyte.
- To distinguish renal tubules (including proximal tubules, distal tubules and thin segments) from collecting ducts.
- To identify macula densa and juxtaglomerular cells from juxtaglomerular apparatus.
- To identify urinary bladder and ureter as organs.

教学目标

- 辨认肾皮质与髓质，肾皮质中的皮质迷路与髓放线。
- 辨认肾小体结构：血管极与小管极，血管球，肾小囊以及足细胞。
- 根据形态特征区别不同分段的肾小管（近端小管、远端小管及细段）与集合管。
- 辨认球旁复合器中的致密斑和球旁细胞。
- 从器官水平辨认膀胱与输尿管。

1.Kidney

Kidney can be divided into outer (or superficial) cortex with dark stain and inner (or deeper) medulla with light stain under microscope with low power objective, which can be easily distinguished because of arcuate arteries and veins traveling between them (Fig. 14-1).

1.肾

低倍镜下可观察到肾脏分为表层深染的皮质和深层浅染的髓质，二者交界处因有较大的弓形动静脉走行而易于区分（图14-1）。

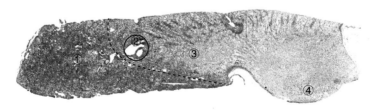

Fig. 14-1   Kidney, from human, by H.E. stain (slide No. Ur1)
图14-1 肾，人，HE染色（切片No. Ur1）

①cortex	①皮质
②arcuate blood vessels	②弓形血管
③medulla	③髓质
④renal papilla	④肾乳头

(1) Kidney cortex

In renal cortex, round renal corpuscles surrounded by convoluted tubules can be seen, which are called cortical labyrinth. Interlobular arteries and veins run in cortical labyrinth. Medullary ray composed of both the straight part of the renal tubules and collecting tubes can be seen among cortical labyrinths (Fig. 14-2).

（1）肾皮质

肾皮质中可见圆形肾小体结构，周围分布有肾小管曲部，称为皮质迷路。皮质迷路中可见小叶间动静脉走行，皮质迷路之间，有肾小管直部和集合管构成的结构，称为髓放线（图14-2）。

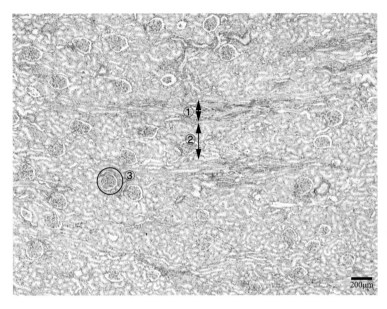

Fig. 14-2　Kidney, from human, by H.E. stain (slide No. Ur1) (×10)

图14-2　肾，人，HE染色（切片No. Ur1）（×10）

①medullary ray　　　①髓放线
②cortical labyrinth　②皮质迷路
③renal corpuscles　③肾小体

Under microscope with high magnification, renal corpuscle is the most distinctive structure of cortex, with glomerulus at its center, which is composed of a tuft of capillaries formed by branches of afferent arterioles. Endothelial cells cannot easily be distinguished from intraglomerular mesangial cells. Outer surface of capillary is coated with cells of visceral layer of Bowman's capsule, i.e., podocytes. The processes of podocytic cytoplasm cannot easily be distinguished in H.E. stain, but podocyte's large, round or oval nuclei with loose chromatin invaginated into the lumen of Bowman's capsule, can easily be identified. Parietal layer of Bowman's capsule is lined with simple squamous epithelium, where Bowman's capsule connecting with proximal convoluted tubules is transitional to simple cuboidal epithelium, i.e., tubular pole (or urinary pole), and where arterioles entering and exiting renal corpuscle is called vascular pole (Fig. 14-3, Fig. 14-4).

高倍镜下，肾小体是肾皮质最明显的结构。肾小体中央为肾血管球，即由入球微动脉分支形成的一丛毛细血管团，肾血管球内皮细胞和球内系膜细胞不易分辨。毛细血管外表面被覆有特化的肾小囊脏层细胞。足细胞，HE染色下足细胞胞质突起不易分辨，但细胞核大，呈圆或椭圆形，染色质疏松，突向肾小囊腔，从而容易辨认。肾小囊壁层被覆一层单层扁平上皮，其与近曲小管连接处上皮移行为单层立方，即小管极（尿极），微动脉进出肾小体的部位称为血管极（图14-3，图14-4）。

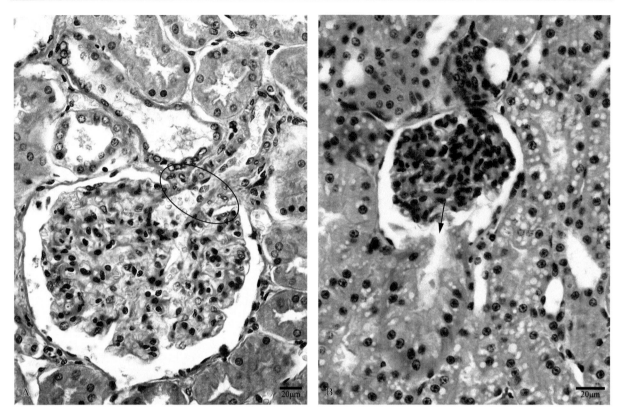

Fig. 14-3　Kidney, from human, by H.E. stain (slide No. Ur1)（×40）

图14-3　肾，人，HE染色（切片No. Ur1）（×40）

A. Vascular pole; B. Tubular pole

A. 血管极；B. 小管极

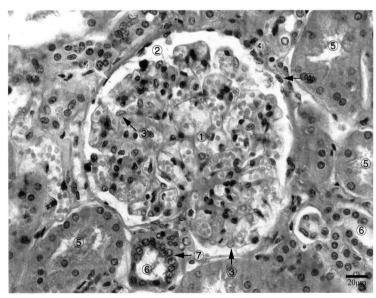

Fig. 14-4　Cortical labyrinth in kidney, from human, by H.E. stain (slide No. Ur1)

图14-4　肾皮质迷路，人，HE染色（切片 No. Ur1）

① glomerulus	① 血管球
② capsular space	② 肾小囊腔
③ podocyte	③ 足细胞
④ simple squamous epithelium parietal layer of Bowman's capsule	④ 肾小囊壁层单层扁平上皮
⑤ proximal convoluted tubule	⑤ 近曲小管
⑥ distal convoluted tubule	⑥ 远曲小管
⑦ macula densa	⑦ 致密斑

Cross-sections of many convoluted tubules surrounding renal corpuscle can be seen, with proximal convoluted tubules as the most numerous in quantity, larger in diameter, and smaller irregular lumen. Their epithelia are composed of large broad cuboidal cells, with strong acidophilic cytoplasm, round nuclei, and sometimes brush borders at their free surface. Distal convoluted tubules are less in number, with regular lumen and smaller cuboidal epithelial cells, so more nuclei can be seen in the section comparing with proximal convoluted tubules. Epithelial cells of distal convoluted tubules have weaker acidophilic cytoplasm than that of proximal convoluted tubules (Fig. 14-4).

Medullary ray includes three types of tubules. Wall structure of the proximal straight tubule (as a component of descending medullar loop) is generally similar to that of proximal convoluted tubule. That of the distal straight tubule (as a component of ascending medullar loop) is similar to that of distal convoluted tubule. Epithelial cells of the collecting tube stain the lightest (or the palest) with a clear demarcation between cells and can easily be distinguished (Fig. 14-5).

肾小体周围可见多个肾小管曲部的横截面，其中近曲小管数量最多，管径大，管腔小而不规则，上皮细胞为大立方形细胞，胞质嗜酸性强，细胞核圆，数量相对少，游离面有时可见刷状缘。远曲小管数量少，管腔规则，立方上皮细胞体积小，因此截面上可见多个细胞核，胞质嗜酸性弱于近曲小管（图14-4）。

髓放线中含有3种小管：近直小管（组成髓袢降支）管壁结构类似近曲小管；远直小管（组成髓袢升支）管壁结构类似远曲小管；集合管上皮细胞染色最浅淡，细胞界限清晰，易于区分（图14-5）。

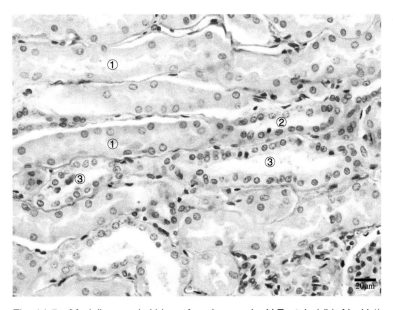

Fig. 14-5　Medullary ray in kidney, from human, by H.E. stain (slide No. Ur1)

图14-5　肾髓放线，人，HE染色（切片No. Ur1）

①proximal straight tubule　　　　　①近直小管
②distal straight tubule　　　　　　②远直小管
③collecting tube　　　　　　　　　③集合管

Epithelium of the distal tubules close to vascular pole of renal corpuscle can be specialized in its sensory function, with higher cells and more densely packed nuclei, referred to macula densa, which is a concentration sensor for sodium ions in tubular fluids. Smooth muscle in the wall of afferent arterioles can be specialized as juxtaglomerular cells with endocrine secretory function, with cells bigger in size, larger and rounded nuclei, loose chromatin, and purplish-blue renin granules can be seen by special histochemical stain (Fig. 14-6). Nuclei of extraglomerular mesangial cells (or Lacis cells) can be found between the macula densa and the juxtaglomerular cells.

肾小体血管极附近的远端小管上皮可发生特化，细胞变高，细胞核排列紧密，称为致密斑，为小管液中钠离子浓度感受器。入球微动脉壁上的平滑肌特化为具有内分泌功能的球旁细胞，其体积大，细胞核大而圆，染色质疏松，特殊染色可见胞质中蓝紫色肾素颗粒（图14-6）。致密斑和球旁细胞间可见球外系膜细胞（Lacis细胞）核。

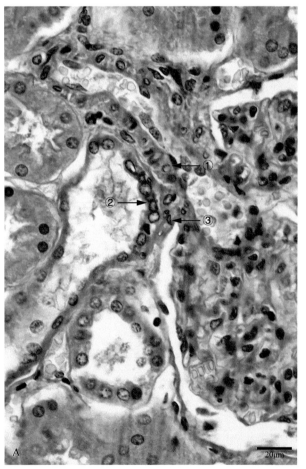
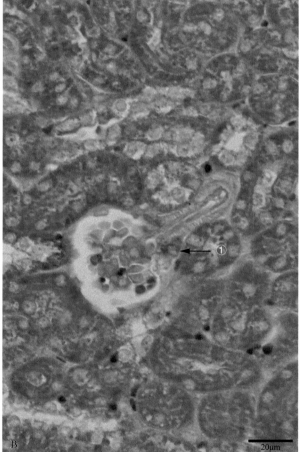

Fig. 14-6　Juxtaglomerular Apparatus (demonstration slide)
图14-6　球旁器（示教切片）

A. Kidney, from human by H.E. stain; B. Kidney, by Bowie stain
①juxtaglomerular cell
②macula densa
③extraglomerular mesangial cell

A. 肾，人，HE染色；B. 肾，Bowie染色
①球旁细胞
②致密斑
③球外系膜细胞

(2) Kidney medulla

Parenchymal components of renal medulla consist of collecting ducts, the straight part of the renal tubule and the thin segment (or limb). The difference between proximal straight tubules and distal straight tubules is similar to that between convoluted ones. Thin segment is the thinnest segment of renal tubule, lined with simple squamous epithelium, similar to the capillary endothelium, but a little bit thicker, without blood cells normally, distinguishable from capillary. Epithelium of collecting ducts is composed of simple cuboidal cells to short-columnar cells, with light stain and clear cellular demarcation (Fig. 14-7).

（2）肾髓质

肾髓质的实质中分布有肾小管直部、细段和集合管。近直小管和远直小管的区别同曲部。细段为肾小管直径最细的一段，被覆单层扁平上皮，但上皮厚度较毛细血管内皮厚，正常情况下不含有血细胞，可借以区分。集合管上皮为单层立方到矮柱状，染色浅，细胞界限清晰（图14-7）。

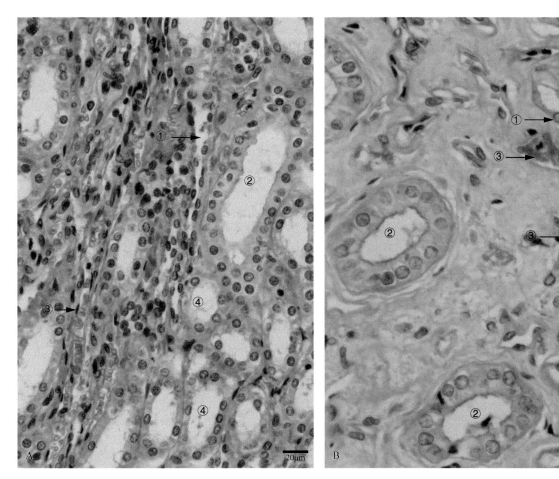

Fig. 14-7   Kidney medulla, from human, by H.E. stain (slide No. Ur1)
图14-7 肾髓质，人，HE染色（切片No. Ur1）

A. Outer medulla; B. Inner medulla
①thin segment
②collecting duct
③blood vessel
④distal straight tubule

A. 外髓；B. 内髓
①细段
②集合管
③血管
④远直小管

In order to observe renal blood vessels, red ink was injected into rabbit kidney before sacrificed. Therefore blood vessels in this slide show red (Fig. 14-8).

为更好显示肾内血管，兔肾血管内注射红墨水后取材制片，血管内均显示红色（图14-8）。

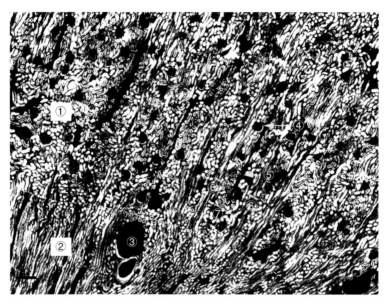

Fig. 14-8　Kidney, from rabbit, intravascular ink injection (demonstration slide)

图14-8　肾，兔，血管注射（示教切片）

①cortex
②medulla
③arcuate blood vessels
④glomerulus
⑤interlobular artery
⑥medullary rays
⑦cortical labyrinth

①皮质
②髓质
③弓形血管
④血管球
⑤小叶间动脉
⑥髓放线
⑦皮质迷路

2.Ureter

Empty ureter has an irregular or asterisk (star-like) lumen with longitudinal mucosa projecting into the lumen. Ureteral wall consists of three layers of mucosa, muscularis and adventitia. Mucosa is composed of transitional epithelium and lamina propria. Muscularis is composed of inner longitudinal and outer circular smooth muscle layers. If the lower ureter is sampled in preparation of the slide, an outer circular smooth muscle layer can be seen in addition to inner longitudinal and circular smooth muscle layers (Fig. 14-9).

2.输尿管

未扩张的输尿管由于黏膜向腔内突起而具有不规则或星形管腔，管壁由黏膜、肌层和外膜3层构成。黏膜由变移上皮和固有层构成。肌层为内纵、外环2层平滑肌，如果切到输尿管下段平滑肌，为内纵、中环、外纵3层（图14-9）。

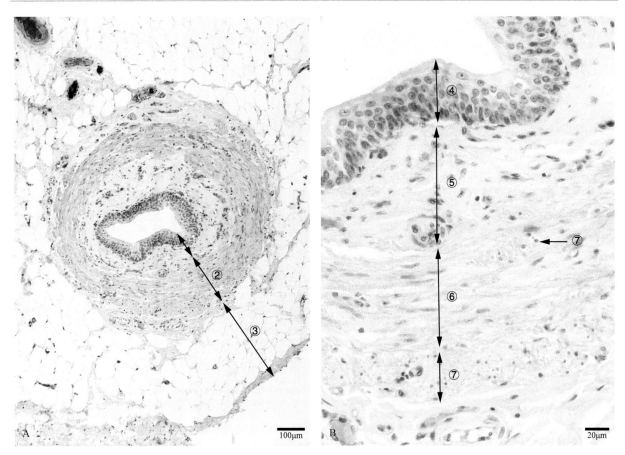

Fig. 14-9　Ureter, from cat, by H.E. stain (slide No. Ur2)
图14-9　输尿管，猫，HE染色（切片No. Ur2）

A.Under low power objective; B.Under high power objective;
①mucosa
②muscularis
③adventitia
④transitional epithelium
⑤lamina propria
⑥circular smooth muscle
⑦longitudinal smooth muscle

A. 低倍镜；B.高倍镜
①黏膜
②肌层
③外膜
④变移上皮
⑤固有层
⑥环行平滑肌
⑦纵行平滑肌

3.Urinary bladder

The wall of urinary bladder is composed of three layers, i.e., mucosa, muscularis and adventitia or serosa, with its mucosa composed of transitional epithelium and lamina propria. The empty urinary bladder has six-to eight-layer cells in epithelial thickness, with larger cell bodies and stronger acidophilic cytoplasm on the superficial layer, called dome cells. When distended, its epithelium becomes thinner and has less layers, with squamous from originally cuboidal (Fig. 1-7 and Fig. 1-8). Its muscularis is thicker and can be divided into not so distinctive three layers of smooth muscles and its adventitia is composed of connective tissue (Fig. 14-10).

3.膀胱

膀胱壁由黏膜、肌层和外膜3层构成。黏膜同样由变移上皮和固有层构成。膀胱空虚时变移上皮厚度为6～8层细胞，表层盖细胞体积大，且嗜酸性较强。膀胱扩张时细胞层数变少，表层盖细胞由立方变成扁平形态（第一章图1-7和图1-8）。肌层厚，可分为不明显的3层平滑肌。外膜为结缔组织（图14-10）。

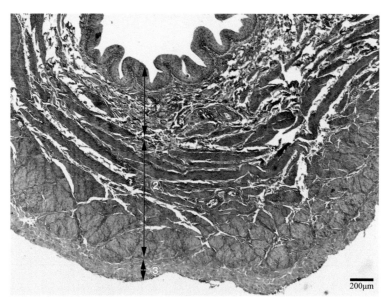

Fig. 14-10　Urinary bladder, from human, by H.E. stain (slide No. Ur3)

图14-10　膀胱，人，HE染色（切片No. Ur3）

①mucosa	①黏膜
②muscularis	②肌层
③adventitia	③外膜

Questions

1.Compare difference in their structure and function between proximal and distal renal tubules.

Characteristics	Proximal tubule	Distal tubule
Number		
Lumen		
Simple cuboidal epithelium		
Spherical nucleus		
Cytoplasm		
Brush border		
Lateral boundary of the cell		
Apical microvilli		
Apical canaliculi and vesicle		
Lateral cell processes		
Basal cell membrane in foldings		
Elongated mitochondria		
Function		

2.How can you identify the juxtaglomerular apparatus under light microscope?

问题

1.比较近端和远端小管形态结构的异同。

特征	近端小管	远端小管
数量		
管腔		
单层立方上皮		
圆形核		
胞质		
刷状缘		
细胞侧面边界		
游离面微绒毛		
游离面管泡		
细胞侧突		
基底面质膜内褶		
长型线粒体		
功能		

2.光镜下如何辨认球旁器？

Chapter 15　EYE and EAR

第十五章　眼　和　耳

Teaching and Learning Objectives

- To identify morphological characteristics of three tunics (or layers) of the wall of eyeball, and especially to distinguish its cornea, iris, ciliary body and retina.
- To identify morphological characteristics of lens.
- To identify morphological characteristics of papilla of optic nerve and central fovea (fovea centralis).
- To identify morphological characteristics of eyelids and the glands in them.
- To distinguish bony labyrinth from membranous labyrinth of inner ears, and to identify morphological characteristics of the maculae of utriculus and sacculus and the cristae ampullares.
- To identify location and structure of the organ of Corti.

教学目标

- 辨认眼球壁3层结构的形态特点，特别是区别角膜、虹膜、睫状体和视网膜的形态。
- 辨认晶状体的形态特点。
- 辨认视神经乳头和中央凹的形态特点。
- 辨认眼睑的形态特点及主要的组成腺体。
- 区别内耳的骨迷路和膜迷路，辨认椭圆囊斑、球囊斑和壶腹嵴的形态特点。
- 辨认螺旋器的位置和结构特点。

1.Eye

First, observe the general topography of eyeball under microscope with low power objective and identify external fibrous layer (cornea and sclera), middle vascular layer (iris, ciliary body and choroid), and inner sensory layer (retina) which communicates with cerebrum through posterior optic nerve; and further identify the lens, pupil, anterior chamber and posterior chamber (Fig. 15-1, Fig. 15-2).

1.眼

首先，低倍镜下观察眼球的整体结构，辨认位于眼球壁外侧的纤维膜（角膜、巩膜）、中层的血管膜（虹膜、睫状体、脉络膜）和内层的视网膜，视网膜通过后部的视神经与大脑相连；之后，再辨认眼球的晶状体、瞳孔、前房和后房（图15-1，图15-2）。

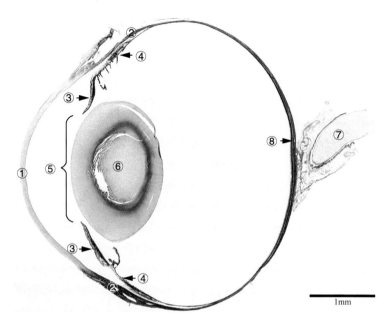

Fig. 15-1　Eye ball, by H.E. stain (slide No. Se1)

图15-1　眼球，HE染色（切片 No. Se1）

① cornea	①角膜
② sclera	②巩膜
③ iris	③虹膜
④ ciliary body	④睫状体
⑤ pupil	⑤瞳孔
⑥ lens	⑥晶状体
⑦ optic nerve	⑦视神经
⑧ choroid and retina	⑧脉络膜和视网膜

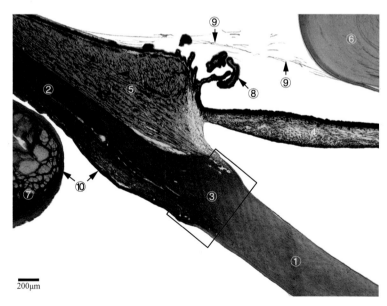

Fig. 15-2　Part of eye ball, by H.E. stain (slide No. Se1)

图15-2　眼球局部，HE染色（切片 No. Se1）

① cornea	①角膜
② sclera	②巩膜
③ limbus cornea	③角膜缘
④ iris	④虹膜
⑤ ciliary body	⑤睫状体
⑥ lens	⑥晶状体
⑦ eyelid	⑦眼睑
⑧ ciliary process	⑧睫状突
⑨ ciliary zonule	⑨睫状小带
⑩ conjunctiva	⑩结膜

Then, study the detailed structure of the eyeball under microscope with higher magnification. Cornea consists of five layers: corneal epithelium, anterior limiting membrane, corneal stroma, posterior limiting membrane, and corneal endothelium. Note that, at the limbus cornea (corneoscleral junction), corneal epithelium is continuing with bulbar conjunctiva, corneal stroma is continuing with sclera, and posterior limiting membrane and corneal endothelium are replaced by trabecular meshwork (a system of irregular endothelium-lined channels). Identify scleral venous sinus (or canal of Schlemm) and trabecular meshwork. Observe the components of ciliary body: ciliary muscles, ciliary processes, ciliary zonule, ciliary epithelium and stroma (Fig. 15-3, Fig. 15-4).

然后在高倍镜下观察眼球的详细结构。角膜由5层构成：角膜上皮、前界膜、角膜基质、后界膜和角膜内皮。注意在角膜缘的部位，角膜上皮和球结膜相连，角膜基质和巩膜相连，后界膜和角膜内皮被小梁网（包被内皮的不规则管网系统）所替代。辨认巩膜静脉窦和小梁网。观察睫状体的组成成分：睫状肌、睫状突、睫状小带、睫状体上皮和基质（图15-3，图15-4）。

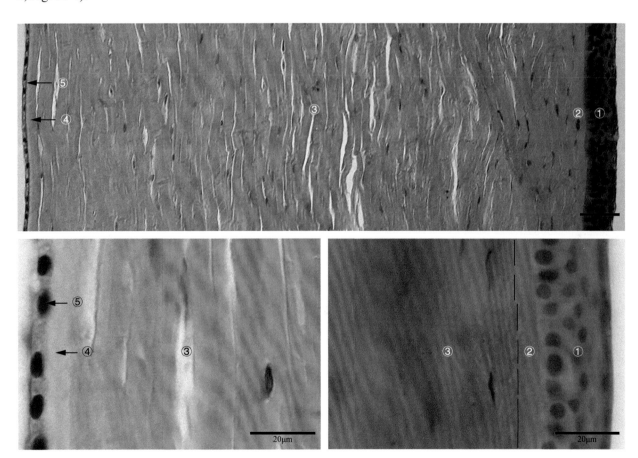

Fig. 15-3   Cornea, by H.E. stain (slide No. Se1)

图15-3   角膜，HE染色（切片No. Se1）

①corneal epithelium
②anterior limiting membrane
③corneal stroma
④posterior limiting membrane
⑤corneal endothelium

①角膜上皮
②前界膜
③角膜基质
④后界膜
⑤角膜内皮

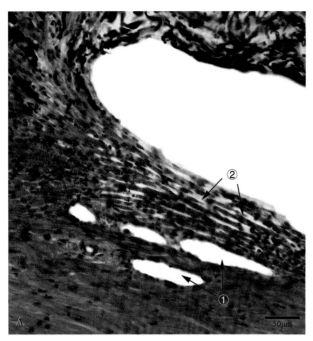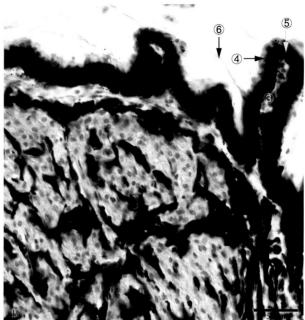

Fig. 15-4　Limbus and ciliary body, by H.E. stain (slide No. Se1)

图 15-4　角膜缘和睫状体，HE 染色（切片 No. Se1）

A. Limbus cornea; B. Ciliary body　　　　　　　　A. 角膜缘；B. 睫状体
①scleral venous sinus　　　　　　　　　　　　　①巩膜静脉窦
②trabecular meshwork　　　　　　　　　　　　　②小梁网
③ciliary process　　　　　　　　　　　　　　　③睫状突
④nonpigmented ciliary epithelium　　　　　　　④睫状体非色素上皮
⑤pigmented ciliary epithelium　　　　　　　　　⑤睫状体色素上皮
⑥ciliary zonule　　　　　　　　　　　　　　　　⑥睫状小带
⑦ciliary muscle　　　　　　　　　　　　　　　　⑦睫状肌

Identify the components of iris: stroma, iris epithelium and sphincter pupillae muscle. Observe the components of lens: capsule, epithelium and fibers (Fig. 15-5).

Note the arrangement and concentration of collagenous fibers in the sclera. The choroid is heavily pigmented, and contains stoma with abundant vessels, choriocapillary lamina and Bruch's membrane. The retina is a ten-layer structure as following (Fig. 15-6) :

(1) Pigment epithelium is the outermost layer of retina, with its basement membrane as component of choroid referred to Bruch's membrane. The other 9 layers refer to neural retina, which extends anteriorly as far as the ora serrata, where it is continuous with the ciliary epithelium (Fig. 15-7).

辨认虹膜的结构：基质、虹膜上皮、瞳孔括约肌。观察晶状体的结构：被膜、上皮和纤维（图 15-5）。

注意巩膜中胶原纤维的排列方式和含量。脉络膜富含色素，包括富含血管的基质、脉络膜毛细血管层和 Bruch 膜。视网膜包含以下 10 层结构（图 15-6）：

（1）色素上皮层，是视网膜的最外层，其基膜构成了脉络膜的 Bruch 膜。视网膜的其他 9 层构成了神经视网膜，它们向前延伸终止于锯齿缘，与睫状体上皮相延续（图 15-7）。

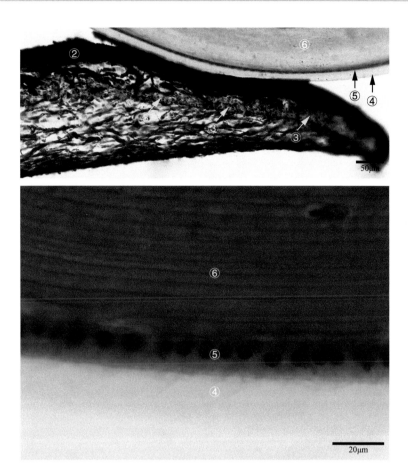

Fig. 15-5　Iris and lens, by H.E. stain (slide No. Se1)

图 15-5　虹膜和晶状体，HE染色（切片 No. Se1）

① iris stroma	① 虹膜基质
② pigmented iris epithelium	② 虹膜色素上皮
③ sphincter pupillae muscles	③ 瞳孔括约肌
④ lens capsule	④ 晶状体被膜
⑤ lens epithelium	⑤ 晶状体上皮
⑥ lens fiber	⑥ 晶状体纤维

(2) Layer of rods and cones.

(3) Outer limiting membrane is a junctional region between photoreceptor cells and specialized ganglial cells called Müller cells, which can not easily be distinguished under light microscope.

(4) Outer nuclear layer consists of nuclei of the rods and cones.

(5) Outer plexiform layer is composed of synapses formed by photoreceptor cells and the bipolar neurons, including the processes of horizontal cells.

(6) Inner nuclear layer contains the cell bodies of bipolar neurons, horizontal cells and amacrine cells.

（2）视杆、视锥层。

（3）外界膜，是Müller细胞和感光细胞之间形成的连接区域，光镜下不易分辨。

（4）外核层，由视杆细胞和视锥细胞的细胞核构成。

（5）外网层，由感光细胞和双极神经元所形成的突触构成，也包含水平细胞的突起。

（6）内核层，由双极神经元、水平细胞和无长突细胞的胞体组成。

(7) Inner plexiform layer is composed of synapses formed by bipolar cells and ganglion cells.

(8) Ganglion cell layer consists of the cell bodies of ganglial cells.

(9) Optic nerve fiber layer is composed of axons of ganglion cells, which converge toward the papilla of optic nerves where they exit from the eyeball (Fig. 15-7).

(10) Inner limiting membrane adjacent to the vitreous body is the innermost layer of retina, which is composed of the mutual junctions among terminal expansions of Müller cells.

The central fovea, the area of clearest vision, is a shallow depression within the retina. It contains only cones and no rods, where ganglionic and inner nuclear layers are spread peripherally (Fig. 15-7).

（7）内网层，由双极神经元和神经节细胞的突触所形成。

（8）神经节细胞层，由神经节细胞的胞体构成。

（9）神经纤维层，由神经节细胞轴突形成的视神经纤维构成，从视神经乳头（图15-7）处离开眼球。

（10）内界膜，紧邻玻璃体，是视网膜的最内层，由Müller细胞的末端膨大相互连接所构成。

中央凹是视网膜中的一个小凹陷，它只有视锥细胞，没有视杆细胞，神经节细胞和内核层都分散于外周，是视网膜视觉最敏锐的区域（图15-7）。

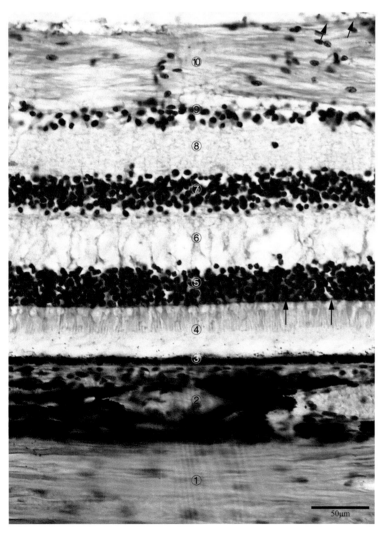

50μm

Fig. 15-6　Retina, by H.E. stain (slide No. Se1)

图15-6　视网膜，HE染色（切片No. Se1）

①sclera	①巩膜
②choroid	②脉络膜
③retinal pigment epithelium	③视网膜色素上皮层
④rod and cone layer	④视杆视锥层
⑤outer nuclear layer	⑤外核层
⑥outer plexiform layer	⑥外网层
⑦inner nuclear layer	⑦内核层
⑧inner plexiform layer	⑧内网层
⑨ganglion cell layer	⑨神经节细胞层
⑩nerve fiber layer	⑩神经纤维层
Arrow: outer limiting membrane; Arrow head: inner limiting membrane	长箭头：外界膜；短箭头：内界膜

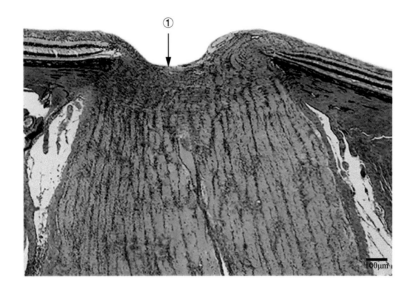

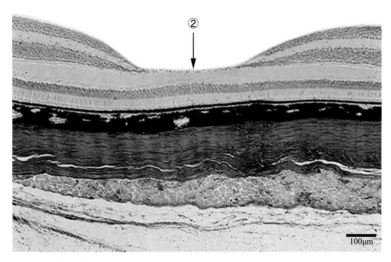

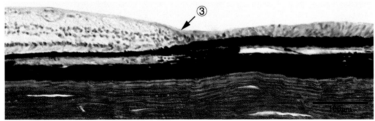

Fig. 15-7　Eyeball, by H.E. stain (demonstration slide)

图 15-7　眼球，HE 染色（示教切片）

①papilla of the optic nerve　　①视神经乳头

②central fovea　　②中央凹

③ora serrata　　③锯齿缘

147

2.Eyelid

The outermost layer of eyelid is skin. That underneath skin is skeletal muscle fibers belonging to the orbicularis oculi, and next to it is tarsal plates which consists of dense fibrous and elastic tissues, with lots of sebaceous glands, i.e., tarsal glands. The innermost layer of tarsal plates is conjunctiva. At the outer rim of eyelid, there are lots of hair follicles for the eyelashes. Those associated with these hair follicles are small sebaceous glands and modified apocrine sweat glands. The former is called the glands of Zeis and the latter the glands of Moll with larger lumen and stronger acidophilic cytoplasm. Near the conjunctiva, lacrimal glands can be seen, which are composed of numerous serous acinic cells (Fig. 15-8, Fig. 15-9).

2.眼睑

眼睑的最外层是皮肤，皮下的骨骼肌属于眼轮匝肌，睑板位于更深层，由致密的纤维和弹性组织构成，内含大量皮脂腺，为睑板腺，睑板的最内层是结膜。在睑缘处，有大量睫毛的毛囊，与之相伴的是小的皮脂腺和顶泌汗腺，前者命名为Zeis腺，后者命名为Moll腺，管腔大，腺细胞嗜酸性强。靠近结膜处可见泪腺，由大量浆液性腺细胞构成（图15-8，图15-9）。

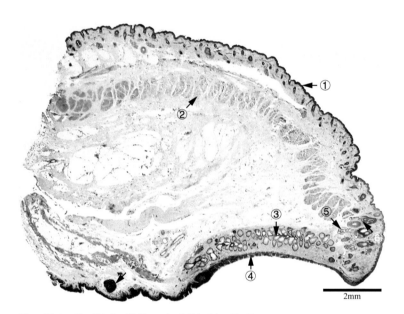

2mm

Fig. 15-8　Eyelid, by H.E. stain (slide No. Se2)
图15-8　眼睑，HE染色（切片No. Se2）

①epidermis	①表皮
②skeletal muscle	②骨骼肌
③tarsal gland	③睑板腺
④conjunctiva	④结膜
⑤Moll gland	⑤Moll腺
⑥Zeis gland	⑥Zeis腺
⑦lacrimal gland	⑦泪腺

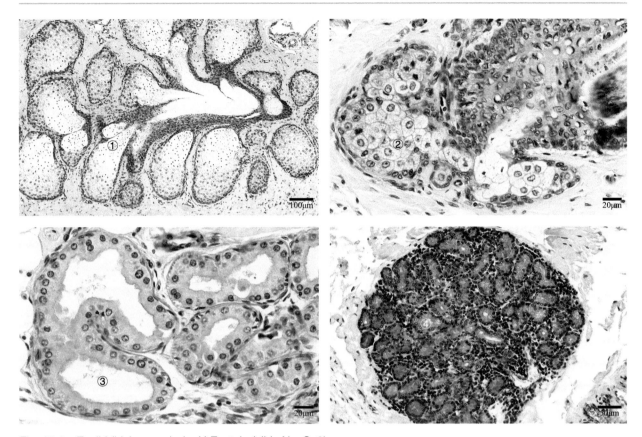

Fig. 15-9   Eyelid (high power) , by H.E. stain (slide No. Se2)
图 15-9   眼睑（高倍），HE 染色（切片 No. Se2）

①tarsal gland
②Zeis gland
③Moll gland
④lacrimal gland

①睑板腺
②Zeis 腺
③Moll 腺
④泪腺

3.Inner ear

Inner ear lies in the petrous portion of temporal bone. A series of canals and small cavities in this bone constitute bony labyrinth. That suspended in the bony labyrinth is membranous labyrinth (endolymphatic system) filled with endolymph. The space between bony labyrinth and membranous labyrinth is filled with perilymph (Fig. 15-10).

3. 内耳

内耳位于颞骨岩部，骨中的小腔隙和小管构成了骨迷路，膜迷路悬吊在骨迷路中，膜迷路中有内淋巴液，膜迷路和骨迷路之间有外淋巴液（图 15-10）。

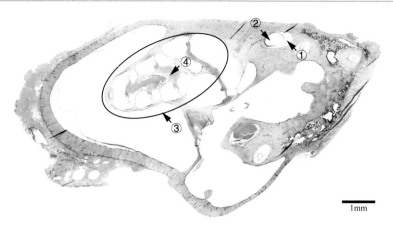

Fig. 15-10　Inner ear, by H.E. stain (slide No. Se3)
图15-10　内耳，HE染色（切片No. Se3）

①bony labyrinth
②membranous labyrinth
③cochlea
④modiolus

①骨迷路
②膜迷路
③耳蜗
④蜗轴

Membranous labyrinth consists of simple squamous epithelium, which is differentiated (or specialized) into hair cells and supporting cells in the cristae ampullae of semicircular ducts or macula utriculi or macula saccule. Surface of the cristae ampullae is covered with colloidal mass (or cupula) which may be very imperfectly preserved during the tissue preparation. Surface of the maculae is covered with an otolithic membrane, a gelatinous membrane composed of gelatinous, glycoprotein mass, i.e., crystal of calcium carbonate (known as otoliths or otoconia) (Fig. 15-11).

膜迷路由单层扁平上皮构成，在半规管壶腹嵴、椭圆囊或球囊斑处特化成毛细胞和支持细胞。壶腹嵴表面覆盖有胶状的壶腹帽，其在制片中可能很难保存下来。斑的表面覆盖有胶状的碳酸钙结晶形成的位砂膜（图15-11）。

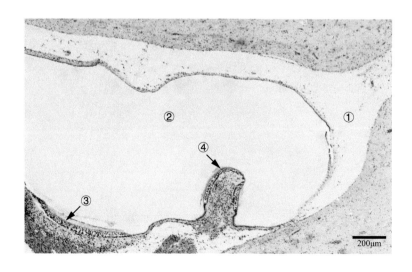

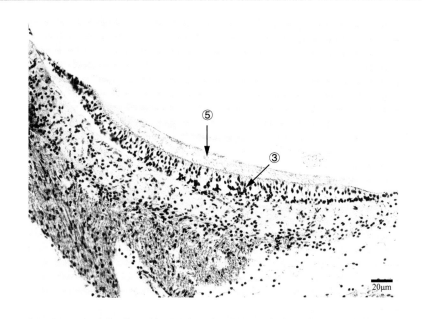

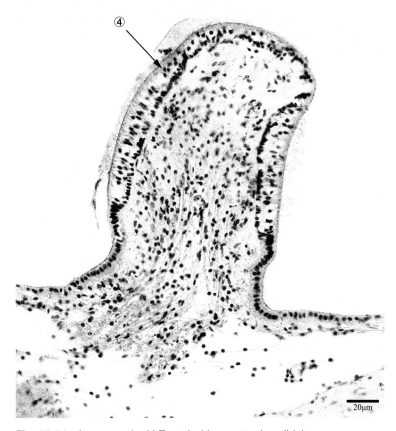

Fig. 15-11　Inner ear, by H.E. stain (demonstration slide)

图15-11　内耳，HE染色（示教切片）

①bony labyrinth　　　　　　　　①骨迷路

②membranous labyrinth　　　　　②膜迷路

③macula of utricle　　　　　　　③椭圆囊斑

④crista ampullaris　　　　　　　④壶腹嵴

⑤otolithic membrane　　　　　　⑤位砂膜

Cochlear duct connects with the saccule, containing endolymph and hearing sensor—the organ of Corti. Cochlear duct is surrounded by two spaces containing perilymph, i.e., the scala vestibule and scala tympani, both of which communicate with each other at the apex of the coiled modiolus through an opening (called the helicotrema). Note the simple squamous epithelium lining in them (Fig. 15-12).

Organ of Corti rests on the basilar membrane composed of a layer of collagenous fibers, with hair cells and

膜蜗管和球囊相连，膜蜗管中有内淋巴，内含听觉感受器——螺旋器，膜蜗管被含有外淋巴的两个腔所包绕，分别是前庭阶和鼓室阶，二者在蜗轴顶端的蜗孔处相连通，观察二者内表面覆盖的单层扁平上皮（图15-12）。

螺旋器位于一层胶原样纤维构成的基底膜上，由毛细胞和支持细胞构成。毛细胞与

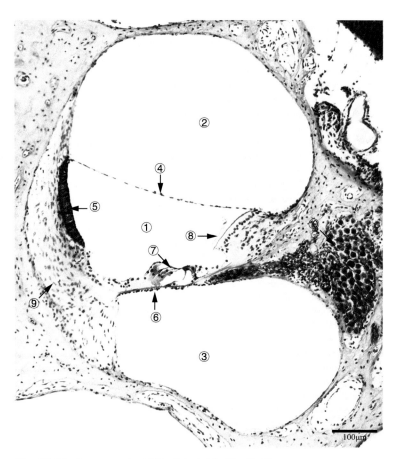

Fig. 15-12   Inner ear, by H.E. stain (slide No. Se3)
图15-12   内耳，HE染色（切片No. Se3）

①cochlear duct	①膜蜗管
②scala vestibule	②前庭阶
③scala tympani	③鼓室阶
④vestibular membrane	④前庭膜
⑤stria vascularis	⑤血管纹
⑥basilar membrane	⑥基底膜
⑦organ of Corti	⑦螺旋器
⑧tectorial membrane	⑧盖膜
⑨spiral ligament	⑨螺旋韧带
⑩spiral ganglion	⑩螺旋神经节

supporting cells. The hair cells are in synaptic contact with classical bipolar neurons, whose bodies make up the spiral ganglion located within the modiolus (a conical pillar of spongy bone surrounded by membranous labyrinth in coiled status). Identify the spiral ganglion. Note the stria vascularis, a vascular area lined with epithelium at outer wall of membranous cochlear duct, involved in secretion of endolymph. Vestibular membrane is a double-layer epithelium (one layer belonging to the cochlear duct and the other to the perilymphatic duct) which separates cochlear duct (scala media) from scala vestibule. Tectorial membrane is a projection extending from inner angle of the cochlear duct, which rests on the surface of hair cells in vivo, but possibly folded back and distorted in preparation of the slide (Fig. 15-13).

位于蜗轴中螺旋神经节内的双极神经元形成突触（蜗轴是一个圆锥柱形的松质骨，耳蜗膜迷路围绕它盘曲而成）。辨认螺旋神经节。观察血管纹，它位于膜蜗管外侧壁被覆上皮中的血管区，产生内淋巴。前庭膜是一个双层上皮膜（一层属于膜蜗管，一层属于外淋巴管），分隔膜蜗管（中间阶）和前庭阶。盖膜是一个从膜蜗管内角伸出的突起，活体状态下盖在毛细胞表面，但制片时可能折叠变形（图15-13）。

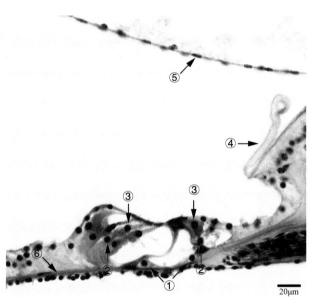
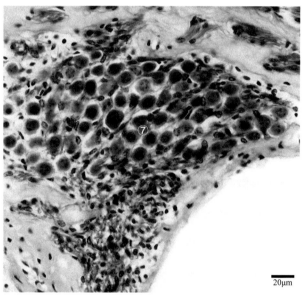

Fig. 15-13   Inner ear, by H.E. stain (slide No. Se3)
图15-13　内耳，HE染色（切片No. Se3）

①pillar cell
②phalangeal cell
③hair cell
④tectorial membrane
⑤vestibular membrane
⑥basilar membrane
⑦spiral ganglion

①柱细胞
②指细胞
③毛细胞
④盖膜
⑤前庭膜
⑥基底膜
⑦螺旋神经节

Questions

Is there any changes in the thickness of the ganglion cell layer throughout the retina?

问题

视网膜中神经节细胞层的厚度有没有改变?

Chapter 16　FEMALE REPRODUCTIVE SYSTEM

第十六章　女性生殖系统

Teaching and Learning Objectives

- To identify ovaries and distinguish varied structures of ovarian cortex, including primordial follicles, primary follicles, secondary follicles, corpus luteum, corpus albicans and interstitial glands.
- To identify oviducts (or fallopian tubes) and distinguish their varied parts.
- To identify uterus and distinguish secretory stage from proliferation stage of endometrium.
- To identify different parts of uterine cervix.
- To identify mammary gland and distinguish its resting and active periods.

教学内容

- 辨认卵巢，识别卵巢皮质中的各个结构，如原始卵泡、初级卵泡、次级卵泡、黄体、白体、间质腺等。
- 辨认输卵管，区分输卵管各个部分。
- 辨认子宫，区分增生期和分泌期的子宫内膜。
- 辨认宫颈，区分宫颈各个部分。
- 辨认乳腺，区分静止期和活跃期的乳腺。

1.Ovaries

(1) Ovarian follicles

The ovaries are oval structure, covered by simple squamous or cuboidal epithelium, referred to ovarian surface epithelium, with a thinner layer of dense connective tissue beneath it, referred to tunica albuginea. The tunica albuginea stains blue in Mallory stain due to its large amount of collagenous fibers (Fig. 16-2). The ovaries are divided into outer cortex and inner medulla. Ovarian medulla is mainly consists of lots of loose connective tissue stroma, with numerous blood and nerves embedded in it. Ovarian cortex is thicker and has numerous ovarian follicles at various stages of development, except lots of stromal components (Fig. 16-1A).

There are three types of ovarian follicles can be recognized in slide No. Fe1:

1) Primordial follicles: ovarian follicles at resting period, located in the superficial ovarian cortex with a primary oocyte of large, rounded and pale-stain nucleus, at the center surrounded by a single layer of flattened follicular cells.

1.卵巢

（1）卵泡

卵巢为椭圆形结构，表面覆盖一层单层扁平或立方的上皮，称为卵巢表面上皮，下方为一薄层结缔组织构成的白膜。白膜中由于有大量胶原纤维的存在，Mallory三色染色时被染成蓝色（图16-2）。卵巢的实质分为外周的皮质和中央的髓质，髓质主要为结缔组织，其中有血管和神经等走行。皮质较厚，除了大量基质成分外，还有大量发育不同阶段的卵泡分布其中（图16-1A）。

切片No. Fe1可识别3种卵泡。

1）原始卵泡：处于静止状态的卵泡，位于皮质浅层。单层扁平的卵泡细胞围绕在中央初级卵母细胞周围，卵母细胞核大而圆，染色浅。

2) Primary follicles: Cytoplasm of flattened ovarian follicular cells is obviously increasing and becoming cuboidal in shape, called granulosa cells, as the primordial follicles begin growing. The granulosa cells proliferate gradually from single layer to multiple layers, with increasing body size, more and more cytoplasm of the oocytes, and an acidophilic homogenous structure, called zona pellucida, surrounds the oocytes.

3) Secondary follicles: Some small spaces appear among granulosa cells and gradually become a larger follicular antrum, as the follicles continue to develop, with follicular fluids aggregated there. Oocytes and granulosa cells around them finally bulge into the antrum to form a small hill-like projection, called the cumulus oophorus. A layer of granulosa cells close to the zona pellucida transforms to tall-columnar from oval-cuboidal in shape, radially arranged, to form the corona radiate. The oocytes are still primary in nature, with continuously increasing cytoplasm. The stroma around ovarian follicles differentiate to form follicular theca (or theca folliculi). The theca cells are characterized by their steroid-secreting function, as capillaries in the inner layer of follicular theca (theca interna) increase (Fig. 16-1B).

Most follicles never reach full maturity but undergo degeneration and atresia, called as the follicles atresia. When the primary follicle atresia takes place, only collapsed zona pellucida leaves behind. When the secondary follicle atresia takes place, the granulosa cells and oocytes degenerate and disappear, the theca cells around the follicle get hypertrophia further, and become to interstitial gland. There are numerous lipid droplets in the cytoplasm of interstitial cells, pale in H.E. stain, with dark and round nuclei centrally located. The residual zona pellucida collapse and is surrounded by interstitial gland cells (Fig. 16-1C). As interstitial glands degenerate, apoptotic cells are phagocytosed by macrophages, and stroma cells proliferate and produce many collagenous fibers to form the corpus albicans, which appears homogeneous, transparent and pink in H.E. stain (Fig. 16-1A), or blue by Mallory trichrome stain (Fig. 16-2).

2）初级卵泡：当原始卵泡开始生长，扁平的卵泡细胞胞质明显增多，变成立方形，被称为颗粒细胞。颗粒细胞具有增殖能力，逐渐从单层变成多层。卵母细胞的胞质也逐渐增多，细胞个体增大。在卵母细胞和颗粒细胞之间出现一层嗜酸性的均质结构，称为透明带。

3）次级卵泡：随着卵泡继续发育，颗粒细胞间出现一些小腔隙，逐渐形成一个大的卵泡腔，卵泡腔里聚集着卵泡液。卵母细胞和周围颗粒细胞突向卵泡腔，形成一个小丘状突起，称为卵丘。紧贴透明带的一层颗粒细胞由立方形变成高柱状，称为放射冠。卵母细胞仍然为初级卵母细胞，胞质在持续增多。环绕在卵泡周围的基质分化形成卵泡膜。卵泡膜内层毛细血管增加，膜细胞具有分泌类固醇类激素细胞的特征（图16-1B）。

多数卵泡会在发育过程中退化、闭锁，称为闭锁卵泡。初级卵泡闭锁后，只留下塌陷的透明带。当次级卵泡闭锁时，颗粒细胞和卵母细胞退化消失，外周的膜细胞进一步肥大，形成间质腺。间质腺细胞胞质内有大量脂滴分布，HE染色浅淡，细胞核圆，深染居中。残留的透明带塌陷，被间质腺细胞包围（图16-1C）。间质腺退化时凋亡的细胞被巨噬细胞吞噬，基质细胞增殖，分泌胶原纤维形成白体，HE染色时白体为均质透明的粉红色（图16-1A），Mallory三色染色则呈蓝色（图16-2）。

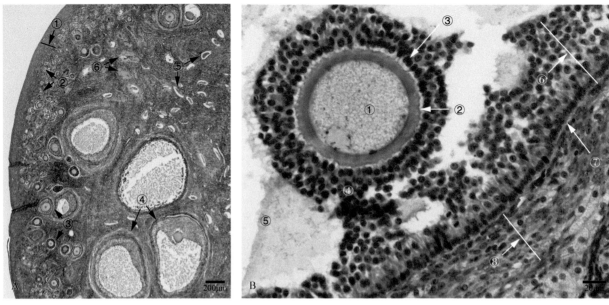

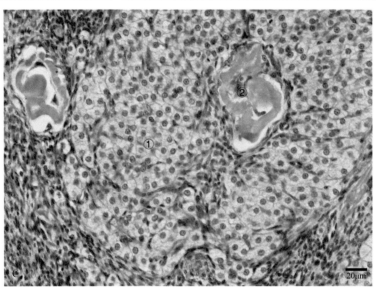

Fig. 16-1　Ovary, from cat, by H.E. stain (slide No. Fe1)
图 16-1　卵巢，猫，HE 染色（切片 No. Fe1）

A. Ovary
①tunica albuginea
②primordial follicles
③primary follicles
④secondary follicles
⑤collapsed zona pellucida
⑥corpus albicans
B. Part of the secondary follicle
①oocyte
②zona pellucida
③corona radiate
④cumulus oophorus
⑤antrum
⑥stratum granulosum
⑦basement membrane
⑧follicular theca
C. Interstitial gland
①interstitial cells
②collapsed zona pellucida

A.卵巢
①白膜
②原始卵泡
③初级卵泡
④次级卵泡
⑤塌陷的透明带
⑥白体
B.次级卵泡局部
①卵母细胞
②透明带
③放射冠
④卵丘
⑤卵泡腔
⑥颗粒层
⑦基底膜
⑧卵泡膜
C.间质腺
①间质腺细胞
②塌陷的透明带

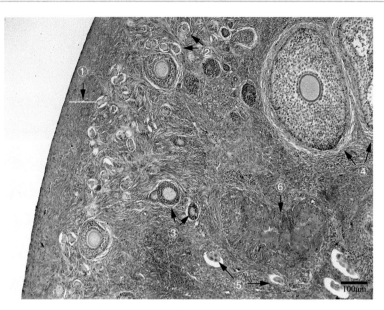

Fig. 16-2　Ovary, from cat, by Mallory trichrome stain (slide No. Fe2)

图16-2　卵巢，猫，Mallory三色染色（切片No. Fe2）

①tunica albuginea	①白膜
②primordial follicles	②原始卵泡
③primary follicles	③初级卵泡
④secondary follicles	④次级卵泡
⑤collapsed zona pellucida	⑤塌陷的透明带
⑥corpus albican	⑥白体

(2) Corpus luteum

When ovarian follicles develop and reach maturity, ovulation begins, both oocytes and the corona radiate ovulate from ovary, and the wall of residual matured follicles collapse, granulosa cells and theca interna cells undergo hypertrophy further to form an endocrine lump, i.e., the corpus luteum (Fig. 16-3). The granulosa lutein cells account for more proportion of the entire corpus luteum, with larger cell body and acidophilic cytoplasm. The theca lutein cells is less in number, small in size, with centrally located dark nucleus and pale-stain cytoplasm, locating around the corpus luteum and near the connective tissue penetrating into the corpus luteum.

（2）黄体

卵泡发育成熟后排卵，卵母细胞和放射冠一同排出卵巢，剩余成熟卵泡的壁塌陷，颗粒细胞和膜细胞进一步肥大，形成一个内分泌团块：黄体（图16-3）。粒黄体细胞在整个黄体中所占比例大，其细胞较大，胞质嗜酸性。膜黄体细胞数量较少，分布于黄体周边和伸入到黄体内的结缔组织周围，膜黄体细胞胞体较小，胞质染色浅淡，细胞核深染。

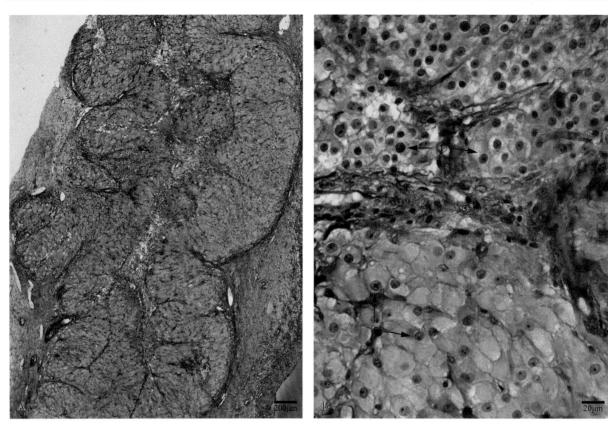

Fig. 16-3　Corpus luteum, from human, by H.E.stain (slide No. Fe9)

图16-3　黄体，人，HE染色（切片No. Fe9）

A. Part of ovary

①corpus luteum

②ovarian stroma

B. Part of corpus luteum

①theca lutein cell

②granulosa lutein cell

③connective tissue

A. 卵巢局部

①黄体

②卵巢基质

B. 黄体局部

①膜黄体细胞

②粒黄体细胞

③结缔组织

(3) Corpus albicans

As the corpus luteum degenerates, lutein cells gradually undergo apoptosis, and their peripheral connective tissue proliferates, with some stromal cells producing lots of collagenous fibers, to form the corpus albicans, appearing homogeneous acidophilic macula in H.E. stain (Fig. 16-4).

（3）白体

当黄体退化时，黄体细胞逐渐凋亡，周围结缔组织增生，基质细胞产生大量胶原纤维，形成白体，HE染色时为均质嗜酸性斑块（图16-4）。

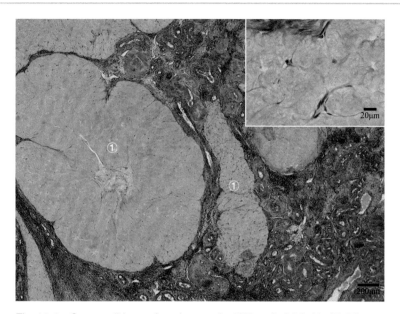

Fig. 16-4　Corpus albicans, from human, by H.E. stain (slide No. Fe10)
图16-4　白体，人，HE染色（切片No. Fe10）

① corpus albicans

Illustration (inserted) : part of corpus albicans under high power objective

①白体

图中图：高倍放大的白体局部

2.Oviducts (fallopian tubes)

Slide No. Fe3 comes from the ampulla of oviducts, taller and larger mucosal folds can be seen in the lumen. The oviduct wall is composed of three layers, i.e., mucosa, muscularis and serosa. The oviduct lines with a simple columnar epithelium, containing two types of cells, i.e., ciliated cells and secretory cells. Cilia can be seen in the apex of ciliated cells, with larger bodies, more cytoplasm and bigger round nuclei. Secretory cells are tall and thin in shape, with elongated and oval nuclei and less cytoplasm. The muscularis is composed of bundles of smooth muscle fibers with lots of interwoven connective tissue and blood vessels. The outermost layer is serosa (Fig. 16-5).

2.输卵管

切片No. Fe3来自输卵管壶腹部，可见管腔中高大的黏膜皱襞。输卵管管壁从内向外依次分为黏膜层、肌层和浆膜层3层。输卵管的上皮为单层柱状上皮，由纤毛细胞和分泌细胞组成。纤毛细胞较大，胞质多，核大，呈椭圆形，细胞顶面可见纤毛；分泌细胞较瘦长，核呈长椭圆形，胞质较少。肌层的平滑肌成束走行，之间交织有大量结缔组织和血管。最外层为浆膜（图16-5）。

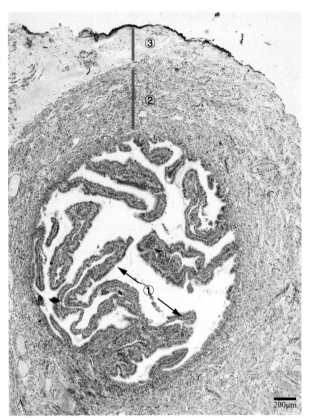

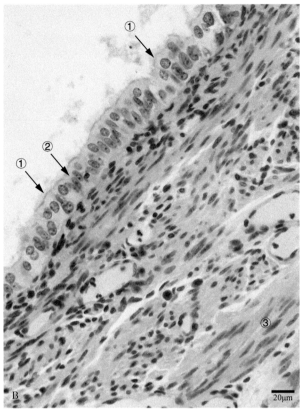

Fig. 16-5　Oviducts, from human, by H.E. stain (slide No. Fe3)

图16-5　输卵管，人，HE染色（切片No. Fe3）

A. Oviducts

①mucosal folds

②muscularis

③serosa

B. Part of oviducts

①ciliated cell

②secretory cell

③smooth muscle bundle

A. 输卵管

①黏膜皱襞

②肌层

③浆膜层

B. 输卵管局部

①纤毛细胞

②分泌细胞

③平滑肌束

3.Uterus

(1) Proliferative phase of endometrium

Under low power objective, distinguish the mucosa, muscularis and serosa of uterus. Uterine muscularis is thick, with interwoven bundles of smooth muscle and connective tissue. Uterine endometrium is composed of epithelium and lamina propria, whereas the former is a simple columnar epithelium consisting of ciliated and secretory cells and dips into the lamina propria forming uterine glands with decreased ciliated cells and increased secretory cells. Lamina propria consists of loose connective tissue with numerous blood vessels. Cells in the uterine stroma and glands appear cyclic alterations

3.子宫

（1）子宫内膜增生期

低倍镜下区分子宫的黏膜层、肌层和浆膜层。子宫肌层很厚，平滑肌束与结缔组织交织分布。子宫内膜由上皮和固有层构成，上皮为单层柱状上皮，包括纤毛细胞和分泌细胞，上皮向固有层凹陷形成子宫腺，子宫腺中纤毛细胞减少，分泌细胞增多。固有层为疏松结缔组织，有丰富的血管分布，基质细胞和子宫腺细胞会随卵巢分泌激素的变化发生周期性改变。子宫内膜还可以分成功能层和基底层，功能层随着激素水平的改变出现增殖、分泌和剥脱等改变，基底层在月经周期不会剥脱，其内的腺

as various hormones secreted from ovaries change. Also, the endometrium can be divided into two layers, i.e., the superficial functionalis and the deeper located basalis. The functionalis emerges changes in proliferation, secretion, slough, and so on as hormone levels alter during menstruation. The basalis is not sloughed during menstruation, with its glands and connective tissue proliferate and thereby regenerate (or repair) the functionalis of endometrium during each menstrual cycle. The endometrium in proliferative phase is thinner with less and more straight glands, proliferated epithelium, densely nuclei, less cytoplasm, as well as proliferative stromal cells (Fig. 16-6).

体和结缔组织增生可以修复剥脱后的子宫内膜功能层。增生期子宫内膜相对较薄，子宫腺数量较少、较直，上皮细胞处于增殖状态，细胞核的密度高，胞质较少。基质细胞也处于增殖状态（图16-6）。

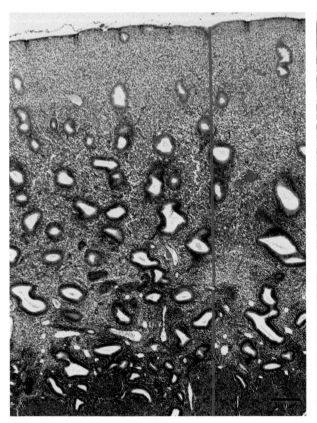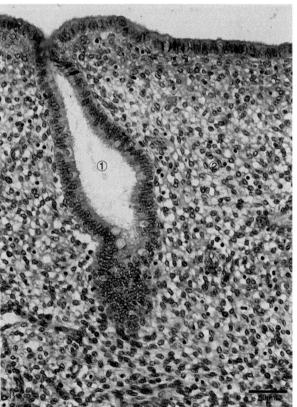

Fig. 16-6　Proliferative phase of uterine endometrium, from human, by H.E. stain (slide No. Fe4)

图16-6　子宫内膜增生期，人，HE染色（切片 No. Fe4）

A. Endometrium

①functional layer of endometrium (functionalis)

②basal layer of endometrium (basalis)

③myometrium

B. Functionalis

①uterine gland

②uterine stroma

A. 子宫内膜

①子宫内膜功能层

②子宫内膜基底层

③子宫肌层

B. 功能层

①子宫腺

②子宫基质

(2) Secretory phase of endometrium

The functional layer of endometrium (functionalis) is thicker in secretory phase of menstruation, with more uterine glands, sawtooth-shaped glandular lumen containing secretion, and more cytoplasm with light-stain. Glycogen synthesized by glandular cells accumulated initially in the lower part of the cells and transferring gradually to the apex of the cells, and finally secreted from the apex. The spiral arteries increase during secretory phase and reach the superficial functionalis (Fig. 16-7).

（2）子宫内膜分泌期

分泌期的子宫内膜功能层较厚，子宫腺数量增多，腺腔呈锯齿状，有分泌物存在。腺细胞胞质多，染色浅淡，细胞合成的糖原最初聚集在核下方，逐渐向细胞顶端转移，最终从细胞顶端分泌出去。分泌期螺旋动脉增加，到达功能层浅层（图16-7）。

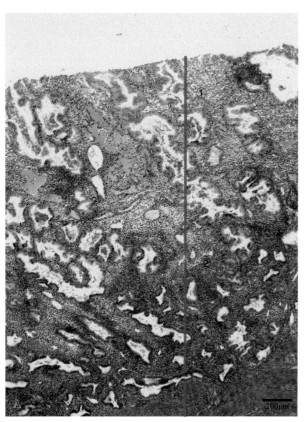
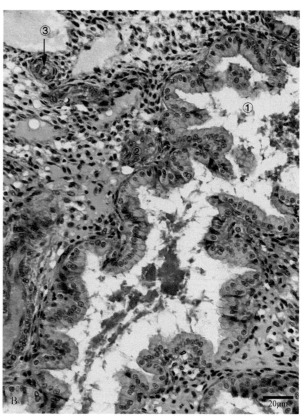

Fig. 16-7　Secretory phase of endometrium, from human, by H.E.stain (slide No. Fe5)
图16-7　子宫内膜分泌期，人，HE染色（切片No. Fe5）

A. Endometrium	A. 子宫内膜
① functional layer of endometrium	①子宫内膜功能层
② basal layer of endometrium	②子宫内膜基底层
③ myometrium	③子宫肌层
B. Functionalis	B. 功能层
① uterine gland	①子宫腺
② uterine stroma	②子宫基质
③ spiral artery	③螺旋动脉

(3) Cervix

The cervix is divided into canal part and vagina part with different types of epithelia, both of which undergo cyclic changes with hormone levels variation, but do not slough during menstruation. Epithelium of cervical canal is tall simple columnar, which goes deep into the lamina propria to form taller and branched tubular gland: cervix glands (Fig. 16-8A). Epithelium of cervical vagina part changes to nonkeratinized stratified squamous directly from simple columnar (Fig. 16-8B).

（3）宫颈

宫颈分为子宫颈管部和宫颈阴道部，两部分上皮类型不同，均会随激素水平变化出现周期性改变，但不会出现周期性剥脱。子宫颈管的上皮为单层柱状上皮，上皮向固有层凹陷，形成高大、有分支的管状腺（图16-8A）。宫颈阴道部上皮直接从单层柱状上皮变为未角化的复层扁平上皮（图16-8B）。

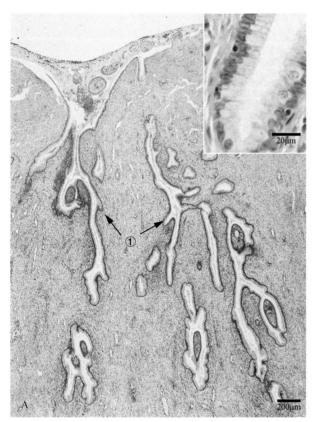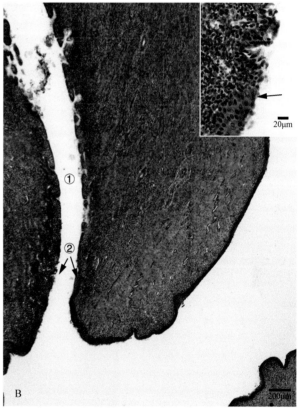

Fig. 16-8　Uterine cervix, from human, by H.E. stain
图16-8　宫颈，人，HE染色

A. Wall of cervical canal (slide No. Fe6)
①cervical gland
Illustration (inserted) Epithelium of cervical gland
B. Transformation zone (demonstration slide)
①cervical canal
②transformation zone
Illustration (inserted) : Epithelium junction

A. 子宫颈管管壁（切片No. Fe6）
①子宫颈腺
图中图：子宫颈腺上皮
B. 上皮移行区（示教切片）
①子宫颈管
②上皮移行区
图中图：移行区局部放大

4.Mammary glands

(1) Resting mammary glands

Observing the slide of mammary glands in resting period under low power objective, lots of connective tissue and adipose cells can be seen. Mammary tissue is grouped together to form lobules, where except connective tissue, terminal duct lobular units can mainly be seen in resting period. Under high power objective, cuboidal epithelium can be seen in the mammary ducts, and myoepithelial cells can also be seen between basement membrane and ductal epithelial cells. Interlobular ducts are surrounded by thicker connective tissue (Fig. 16-9).

4.乳腺

（1）静止期乳腺

低倍镜下观察静止期乳腺切片，可见大量结缔组织和脂肪细胞，乳腺组织形成小叶，静止期小叶内除了结缔组织外主要为终末导管结构。高倍镜可见导管上皮为立方形，基底膜与导管上皮细胞之间还可见肌上皮细胞。小叶间导管有较厚结缔组织包绕（图16-9）。

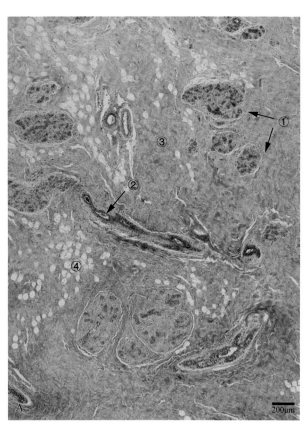
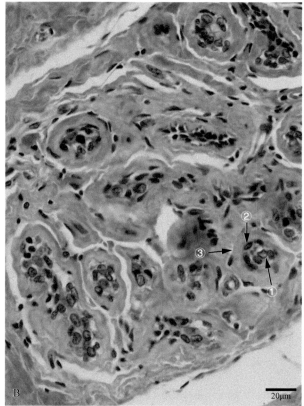

Fig. 16-9　Resting mammary gland, from human, by H.E.stain (slide No. Fe7)

图16-9　静止期乳腺，人，HE染色（切片No. Fe7）

A. Mammary gland	A. 乳腺
①lobule of mammary gland	①乳腺小叶
②interlobular duct	②小叶间导管
③connective tissue	③结缔组织
④adipose tissue	④脂肪组织
B. Lobule of mammary gland	B. 乳腺小叶
①epithelium of intralobular duct	①小叶内导管上皮
②myoepithelial cell	②肌上皮细胞
③basement membrane	③基底膜

(2) Lactating (or active) mammary glands

Entering lactating (or active) period, mammary acini increase leading to mammary lobules enlarged obviously, and interlobular connective tissue and fat decrease. Alveolar cells of the lactating mammary glands synthesize numerous milk and lipid droplets which accumulate in the lumen of acini, and alveolar cells that synthesize milk appear cuboidal or columnar in shape and become squamous after lactation, with dilated lumen of intralobular ducts and milk accumulated in it (Fig. 16-10).

（2）分泌期乳腺

乳腺进入活跃期后，腺泡大量增加，使乳腺小叶明显扩大，小叶间的结缔组织和脂肪减少。分泌期的乳腺，腺泡细胞合成大量乳汁，分泌物聚集在腺泡腔内，合成乳汁的腺泡细胞呈立方或柱状，分泌后的腺泡细胞呈扁平状。小叶内导管腺腔大，常有乳汁聚积（图16-10）。

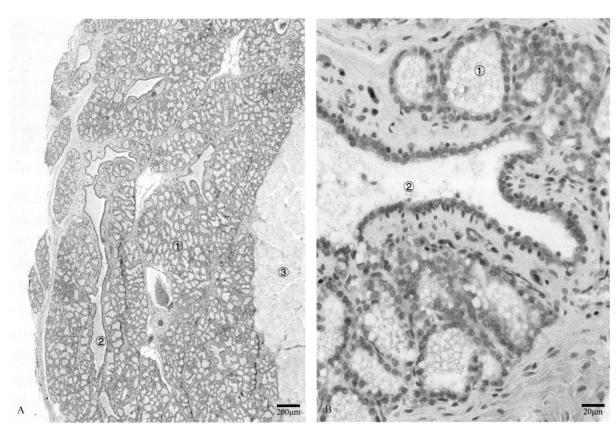

Fig. 16-10　Lactating mammary glands, from dog, by H.E. stain (slide No. Fe8)

图16-10　分泌期乳腺，狗，HE染色（切片No. Fe8）

A. Mammary gland
①lobule of mammary gland
②interlobular duct
③skeletal muscle
B. Lobule of mammary gland
①acinus
②intralobular ducts

A. 乳腺
①乳腺小叶
②小叶间导管
③骨骼肌
B. 乳腺小叶
①腺泡
②小叶内导管

Questions

1.What is the difference in their origin, structure and function between the corpus luteum and interstitial gland?

2.How to distinguish the oviducts from the uterus, the deferent duct and other tubular organs?

问题

1.黄体与间质腺的来源、结构和功能有何不同？

2.输卵管如何与子宫、输精管及其他管状器官区别？

Chapter 17   MALE REPRODUCTIVE SYSTEM
第十七章　男性生殖系统

Teaching and Learning Objectives

- To identify morphological characteristics of interstitial cells (Leydig cells), myoid cells, various spermatogenic cell types and Sertoli cells in the seminiferous tubule of the testis.
- To identify histological structure of tubuli recti and rete testis, and distinguish structural difference of efferent duct from epididymal duct.
- To identify histological structure of the prostate, ductus deferens, seminal vesicle and penis.

教学目标

- 辨认睾丸间质细胞、肌样细胞以及曲细精管中不同种类生精细胞和支持细胞的形态特点。
- 辨认直精小管和睾丸网的组织学结构，区分输出小管和附睾管。
- 辨认前列腺、输精管、精囊腺和阴茎的组织结构。

1.Testis and epididymis

(1) Testis

The testis is covered by a relatively thick connective tissue capsule, i.e., the tunica albuginea. Identify the tunica albuginea of the testis, with its outer surface lined with a simple squamous epithelium-mesothelium (Fig. 17-1).

1.睾丸和附睾

（1）睾丸

睾丸被覆相对较厚的结缔组织被膜——白膜。辨认睾丸的白膜，其外表面贴附有单层扁平上皮构成的间皮（图 17-1）。

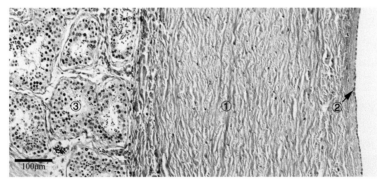

Fig. 17-1   Testis, by H.E. stain (slide No. Ma1)
图 17-1　睾丸，HE 染色（切片 No. Ma1）

①tunica albuginea	①白膜
②mesothelium	②间皮
③seminiferous tubule	③曲细精管

Identify varied types of spermatogenic cells in slide No. Ma1, i.e., spermatogonia, primary spermatocytes, spermatids and spermatozoa within the seminiferous tubules. The spermatogonia are located at the base of seminiferous epithelium, with the primary spermatocytes above them. The primary spermatocytes are the largest cells of the spermatogenic lineage and are characterized by the presence of chromosomes. The secondary spermatocytes are difficult to find in the slide because of their shorter life span, so no need to look for them in your own slides. The round spermatids are located either at the surface of seminiferous epithelium or close to it, with round nuclei and smaller than spermatocytes. During spermiogenesis both nucleus and cytoplasm of the spermatid become elongated, with extremely condensed chromatin and darkly-stained. Cytoplasm can not easily be discerned in matured spermatozoa (Fig. 17-2). Identify the head and tail of spermatozoa (Fig. 17-3).

在切片No. Ma1上辨认不同类型的生精细胞，如位于曲细精管中的精原细胞、初级精母细胞、精子细胞和精子。精原细胞位于生精上皮的基底部，其上为初级精母细胞，初级精母细胞是生精细胞中最大的细胞，细胞内可见染色体是它的特点。次级精母细胞的存在时间很短，所以切片中罕见，无须在切片中寻找它。圆形精子细胞位于或者靠近生精上皮的表面，核圆，比精母细胞小。在精子形成过程中，精子细胞的核和胞质都变长，核染色质极度浓缩，染色很深。成熟精子的胞质不易辨认（图17-2）。辨认精子的头和尾（图17-3）。

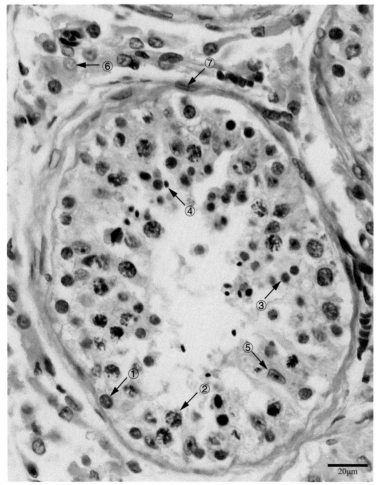

Fig. 17-2　Testis, by H.E. stain (slide No. Ma1)

图17-2　睾丸，HE染色（切片No. Ma1）

①spermatogonium	①精原细胞
②primary spermatocyte	②初级精母细胞
③spermatid	③精子细胞
④spermatozoon	④精子
⑤Sertoli cell	⑤支持细胞
⑥Leydig cell	⑥间质细胞
⑦myoid cell	⑦肌样细胞

Identify Sertoli cells within the seminiferous tubules, with oval or irregular nuclei, prominent nucleoli and pale chromatin. Their cytoplasm is extensive but difficult to discern.

Identify the interstitial cells of testis (or Leydig cells) which lie in the interstitium between seminiferous tubules possibly in solitary, but more common lie in cluster, with large body, polygonal in shape, acidophilic cytoplasm. Note numerous blood vessels around the interstitial cells.

辨认曲细精管中的支持细胞，它的细胞核呈卵圆形或者不规则形，染色浅，核仁明显。支持细胞的胞质很多，但不易分辨。

辨认间质细胞（Leydig细胞），它们可以单个分布于曲细精管之间的间质部位，但更常见的是成群分布，细胞大，多角形，胞质嗜酸性。注意细胞周围有很多血管。

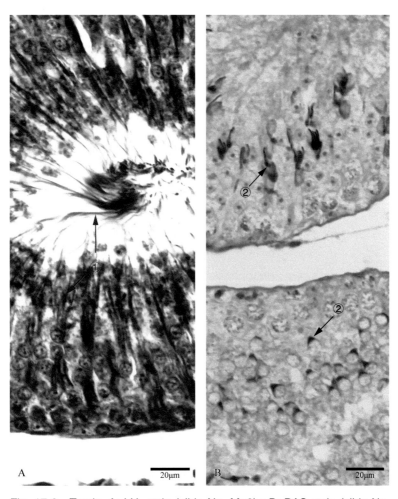

Fig. 17-3   Testis, A: I.H. stain (slide No. Ma2) ; B: PAS stain (slide No. Ma3)

图17-3   睾丸，A：铁苏木精染色（切片No. Ma2）；B: PAS染色（切片No. Ma3）

①tail of the spermatozoa   ①精子尾
②acrosome   ②顶体

(2) Tubuli recti and rete testis

The seminiferous tubules converge toward the posterior dorsal aspect of the testis where they empty into an anastomotic network of rete testis via straight tubules (tubuli recti). Epithelium of the rete testis is simple cuboidal, which locates in the mediastinum of testis (Fig. 17-4).

（2）直精小管和睾丸网

曲细精管在睾丸背侧通过直精小管与睾丸网相连，后者位于睾丸纵隔内，其上皮是单层立方上皮（图17-4）。

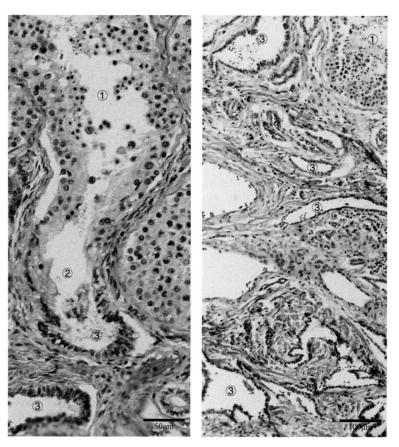

Fig. 17-4　Testis, by H.E. stain (demonstration slide)
图17-4　睾丸，HE染色（示教切片）

①seminiferous tubule　　　　①曲细精管
②tubuli recti　　　　　　　②直精小管
③rete testis　　　　　　　　③睾丸网

(3) Epididymis

Identify the efferent ducts of the epididymis on the slide No. Ma1, which form the head of epididymis, alternately arranged with taller and shorter columnar epithelial cells, causing scallop (or saw-tooth) appearance in the luminal surface. The convoluted epididymal ducts make up the body and tail of the epididymis, with pseudostratified, taller and uniform, columnar epithelial cells with stereocilia extending to the regular luminal surface without undulation. Smaller basal cells locate closer to the basement membrane. Smooth muscle cells surround the efferent ducts and epididymal ducts (Fig. 17-5).

（3）附睾

在切片 No. Ma1 上辨认输出小管，其构成附睾头，管腔由高柱状与低柱状上皮细胞相间排列而成，导致管腔面呈锯齿状。附睾管构成附睾的体部和尾部，由假复层柱状上皮构成，伸达腔面的细胞呈高柱状，整齐划一，其表面有伸入腔面的静纤毛；管腔面很规则；小的基细胞紧邻基底膜分布；平滑肌细胞环绕着输出小管和附睾管（图 17-5）。

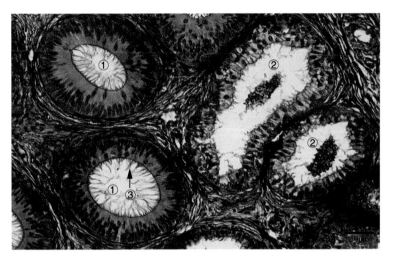

Fig. 17-5　Epididymis, by H.E. stain (slide No. Ma1)
图 17-5　附睾，HE染色（切片 No. Ma1）

①epididymal duct	①附睾管
②efferent duct	②输出小管
③stereocilia	③静纤毛

2.Ductus (vas) deferens

Identify the ductus deferens within the spermatic cord. Note that its epithelium resembles that of the epididymal duct, but due to contraction of smooth muscle in the wall, its mucosa protrudes into the lumen forming much longitudinal, irregular folds. Smooth muscles in the wall are very thick, comprised of three layers of inner longitudinal, intermediate circular and outer longitudinal muscles. Identify striated muscle (cremaster muscle), spermatic artery, nerves and pampiniform plexus of veins surrounding the spermatic artery. Abundant, irregularly oriented smooth muscles line in the venous wall (Fig. 17-6).

2.输精管

辨认位于精索中的输精管，注意其上皮类似于附睾管上皮，但由于管壁平滑肌的收缩，导致黏膜突入管腔形成很多纵行的不规则皱襞。其管壁平滑肌非常厚，由内纵、中环、外纵3层构成。辨认横纹肌（睾提肌），睾丸动脉、神经和环绕着睾丸动脉的蔓状静脉丛。静脉壁有大量不规则排列的平滑肌细胞（图17-6）。

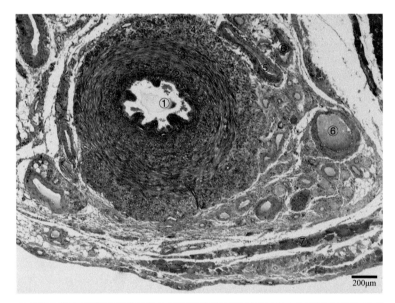

200μm

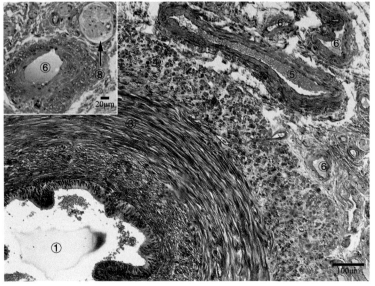

100μm

20μm

Fig. 17-6　Ductus (vas) deferens, by H.E. stain (slide No. Ma4)

图17-6　输精管，HE染色（切片No. Ma4）

①ductus deferens	①输精管
②inner longitudinal smooth muscle layer	②内层纵行平滑肌
③intermediate circular smooth muscle layer	③中层环行平滑肌
④outer longitudinal smooth muscle layer	④外层纵行平滑肌
⑤spermatic artery	⑤睾丸动脉
⑥pampiniform plexus of veins	⑥蔓状静脉丛
⑦cremaster (muscle)	⑦睾提肌
⑧nerve	⑧神经

3.Seminal vesicle

Seminal vesicle is a single, highly coiled sac, with a series of unconnected lumen in the slide. Epithelium of the lumen varies in its thickness, and consists of round cells in the basal layer and a more superficial layer of cells ranging from cuboidal to shorter columnar in shape. Note the stained secretory material in the lumen and also the considerable amount of smooth muscle cells in its wall (Fig. 17-7).

3.精囊腺

精囊腺是一条单一的、高度盘曲的囊管，在切片上显得其管腔并不连通。管腔上皮厚度不均，由基底层的圆形细胞和表层的细胞构成，其形状从立方到低柱状不等。注意精囊腺管腔内染色的分泌物，以及其管壁中大量的平滑肌细胞（图17-7）。

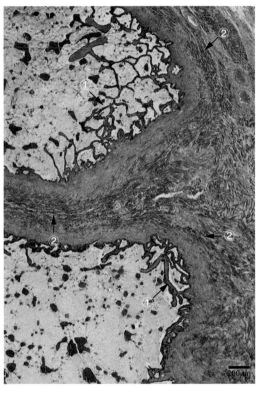
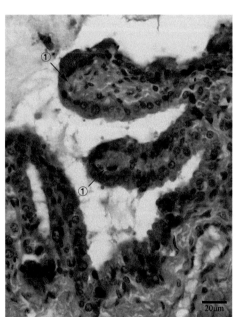

Fig. 17-7   Seminal vesicle, by H.E. stain (slide No. Ma5)

图17-7   精囊腺，HE染色（切片No. Ma5）

①mucosal fold
②smooth muscle

①黏膜皱襞
②平滑肌

4.Prostate

Prostate is made up of numerous small saccular glands. Its epithelium is quite variable in appearance, from simple cuboidal to low columnar. Note that much smooth muscle cells scatter in the stroma. Lamellated concretions of the prostate can be seen within the glandular lumen (Fig. 17-8).

4.前列腺

前列腺由大量的小囊状腺构成，上皮从单层立方到低柱状不等。注意基质中有很多散在的平滑肌细胞。在腺腔中可见前列腺凝固体（图17-8）。

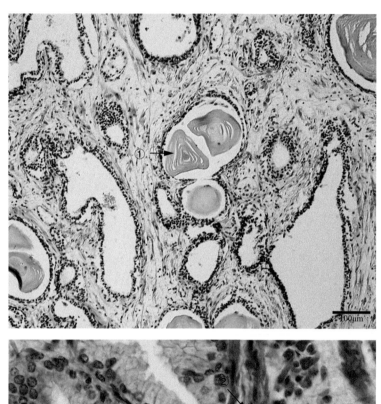

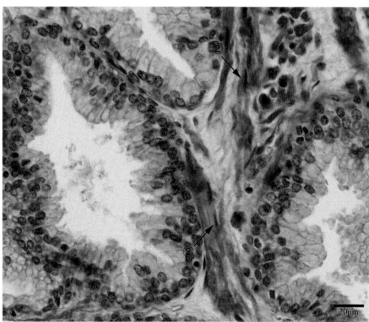

Fig. 17-8　Prostate, H.E. stain (slide No. Ma6)

图 17-8　前列腺，HE 染色（切片 No. Ma6）

①prostatic concretions　　　　　①前列腺凝固体
②smooth muscle　　　　　　　②平滑肌

5.Penis

The penis consists of erectile tissue in the form of a pair of dorsally situated, cylindrical bodies, the corpora cavernosa penis, and a single ventrally located cylindrical body, the corpus cavernosum urethrae (corpus spongiosum), in which the spongy part of the urethra is embedded. All of them are each surrounded by a dense, fibroelastic layer, the tunica albuginea. Erectile tissue contains numerous wide, irregularly shaped venous cavernous spaces lined with endothelium and surrounded by trabeculae with smooth muscle and connective tissue (Fig. 17-9).

5.阴茎

阴茎由一对位于背侧的、圆柱形阴茎海绵体和一个位于腹侧、含尿道的尿道海绵体组成，海绵体均含勃起组织。致密的纤维弹性组织形成白膜，环绕着每一个海绵体。勃起组织含有大量宽的、不规则形状的、覆盖内皮的静脉窦，其周围环绕着平滑肌和结缔组织形成的小梁（图17-9）。

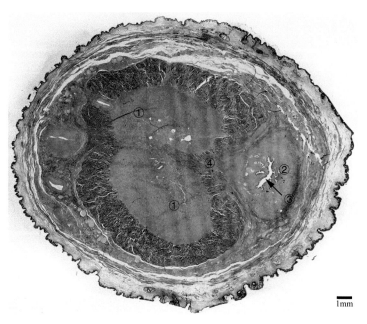
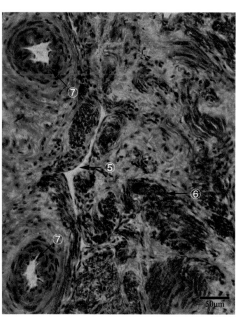

1mm

50μm

Fig. 17-9   Penis, by H.E. stain (slide No. Ma7)
图 17-9   阴茎，HE 染色（切片 No. Ma7）

①corpora cavernosa of the penis
②corpus spongiosum
③penile urethra
④tunica albuginea
⑤venous cavernous space
⑥smooth muscle of the trabeculae
⑦helicine artery

①阴茎海绵体
②尿道海绵体
③尿道阴茎部
④白膜
⑤静脉窦
⑥小梁中的平滑肌
⑦螺旋动脉

Epithelium of the penile urethra is pseudostratified columnar in nature, with its mucosa protruding into its lumen to form prominent longitudinal folds, causing an irregular luminal surface. Also, its epithelium protrudes outwards forming glandular structure in the recesses between those folds, which secrete mucus (or mucin), i. e. the urethral gland (Fig. 17-10).

尿道阴茎部上皮是假复层柱状上皮，其黏膜突入管腔形成纵行皱襞，导致管腔不规则。在皱襞的隐窝内，上皮外凸形成腺样结构，分泌黏液，称为尿道腺（图17-10）。

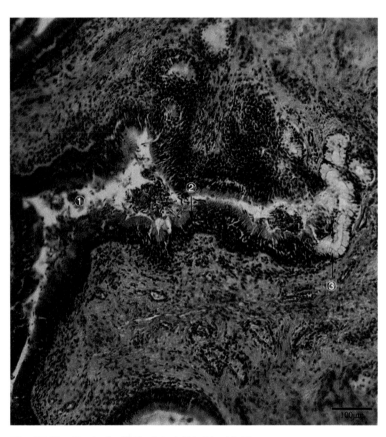

Fig. 17-10　Penis, by H.E. stain (slide No. Ma7)
图17-10　阴茎，HE染色（切片No. Ma7）

①penile urethra
②pseudostratified columnar epithelium
③urethral gland

①尿道阴茎部
②假复层柱状上皮
③尿道腺

Questions

How to distinguish the efferent duct from the epididymal duct in the light microscope?

问题

如何在光镜下区分输出小管和附睾管？